SKINNYCHEATS

THE TRAINERS
SECRETS

"Looking good is the best revenge."

Tony Curtis

SKINNYCHEATS

THE TRAINERS
SECRETS

Ann Macklin

ISBN 978-154257197
ISBN 151425719X

CONTENTS

Part I

Reasons For Writing

I woke up fat one morning -- really. I simply woke up, looked at myself, and I kid you not, during the night I had mysteriously gained almost forty pounds!

I didn't take this well.

As a certified trainer, working in wellness and fitness for more than twenty years, how was I supposed to face my colleagues and clients? How was I supposed to pour myself into spandex? Worse, as I scanned my very evident belly, how was I supposed to face myself?

To be fair to myself, I'd had a pretty rough six months: knee surgery and a fractured foot, followed by a broken foot and a badly sprained ankle. My activity levels dropped, but my eating didn't change a bit. The result? You guessed it – those forty "instant" pounds.

There was no magic involved. I'd simply lost muscle mass and stored up the fat and calories I hadn't burned off. The problem was that I work in an image conscious business. I had to do better – and I had to do it fast.

SKINNYCHEATS
The Trainers Secrets

I was going to have to diet. I didn't begin with the intentional cheat. I just needed to diet, but the thing about diets is that they tend to deprive us of the foods we love. I don't like deprivation any more than anyone else does, but you've got to do what you've got to do.

First week, I drank the water, ate the vegetables, the chicken, and the fish. I lost one pound. Week two, I drank the water, ate the vegetables, the chicken, and the fish. I lost nothing. Week three, I drank the water, ate the vegetables, the chicken, and the fish. I lost one pound. Week four, I drank the water, ate the vegetables, the chicken, the fish, a bagel with cream cheese, a muffin, some frozen yogurt (because it tasted good), and a bag of popcorn. I lost five pounds.

Okay. I lost seven pounds in a month *after* I added some serious carbohydrates? Carbohydrates that tasted good? I lost five of those pounds in *one* week? AND I was feeling *GREAT*! Lots of energy, ready to restart my workouts – I was ready to try it again. I gave it a second week: drank the water, ate the vegetables, the chicken, the fish, fruit every day, and a muffin. I lost three more pounds.

Not bad, huh? Ten pounds gone in five weeks – but more noticeably, eight of those pounds were dropped in TWO weeks. Those eight pounds made a quick and serious dent in the forty pounds I'd gained. That got me thinking, and sent me back to information I've compiled over my twenty-plus years in the wellness/fitness industry.

There were all of those really good and specific reasons that you can find on television and any website or magazine you might choose. Things like the epidemic of obesity in this country, the rise of hypertension, heart attacks, strokes, and osteoarthritis.

SKINNYCHEATS
The Trainers Secrets

Weight control is a large part of the pain management plan for people with bone and joint related issues. As fitness and health professionals, we're trained to avoid "fad" dieting, and the reasons for avoidance make sense, but the pain in my knees made it personal. I looked for ways to make a difference – fast. Yes, I looked for the Skinny Cheats, and the results of my search are within the pages of this book.

This book contains no actual medical plans. I'm not a doctor. What I am is a fitness professional with more than twenty years experience, and based on that experience, I can promise you that anything eaten in excess will increase your body mass and ultimately, your body fat. I can promise you that anything eaten in moderation and combined with a regular plan of aerobic exercise and strength training will help you to attain the slimmer leaner body you're looking for. I can also promise that if you can't see a reward to your effort, you won't stick to any kind of eating plan – no matter how "healthy" it claims to be.

This is the place where I remind you of two important things: First, check with your doctor before you begin any diet or extreme change in eating plans. Second, don't forget that no matter what a diet promises, you will still have to include a regular program of strength training and aerobic exercise to maintain your weight loss progress.

Ever notice that almost every diet and every diet supplement on the market recommends exercise and a caloric intake of approximately 1200 calories per day? Wonder why they can assure you that their particular brand of magic will work – if you follow their "sensible" 1200 calorie eating plan? It works because most people are eating in excess of 2,000 calories a day.

SKINNYCHEATS
The Trainers Secrets

It takes 3500 calories to equal one pound of fat. Doing the math, you can readily see that if you eliminate those extra calories, you drop the pounds. Fewer calories in, and the pounds HAVE to come off!

One of the reasons you picked up this book was because you needed some FAST help. Maybe you need a push to get you headed in the right direction. Maybe you need to see some immediate and measurable progress – just so you'll know that your goal is attainable. Whatever your immediate need, the diets you'll find in this book are going to encourage you to take in less than your usual number of calories.

Used for periods of three to twenty-one days, none of these eating patterns will kill your metabolic rate. In fact, most of them will leave you with enough extra energy and encouragement that you'll find yourself likely to dust off that gym membership card and check out a class, lift a few weights, take a swim, or a nice long walk.

So, let's get you motivated by jump-starting your eating plan. Review the diets that have been included in this book, then choose the plan that will work best with your lifestyle and personal tastes – sorry, we left the Chocolate Diet out. We've called them by their popular names, so you will note several that you've already heard of.

Look for the nutrition plates associated with the soup-based diets. They'll tell you what vitamins and minerals the meals supply. Look for the Dieter Notes with each diet. They'll tell you what to look for in terms of how quickly you can expect to see results, average pounds lost, and energy levels.

When making the transition from any of these diets, back to "regular" eating, remember that if you go back to the habits that caused you to gain the weight in the first place, you will regain it. Working with and coming off any of these plans, remember to:

- Watch your portion sizes.

- Eat all things in moderation. Your body is going to require protein, carbohydrates, and fats. No lifelong plan will eliminate any of these.

- Eat regular small meals (4 – 6 per day, snacks included).

- Drink LOTS of water (64 – 128 ounces per day).

- Include strength training in your exercise program. Aerobic exercise burns calories for every minute that you're exercising. Strength / resistance / weight training builds the muscle that will burn calories 24 hours a day – even while you're sleeping!

Think of this book as a tool in your basic body arsenal – a resource containing information you'll need to fine-tune and maintain the weight that's best for you.

Diet Myths

Okay, you picked up this book because you're ready for a change. You picked up this book because you need a jumpstart on weight loss. And now, you feel guilty about sneaking around – cheating, if you let some people tell it. Here you are, about to try a diet that every magazine on the rack, everybody at the gym, practically every show on TV, and the folks at your job have all promised will fail – miserably.

They've promised that your metabolic rate will crash and that you will never be able to rev it up again. On top of that promise, you're probably the recipient of a lot of other really *wrong*, though well-meaning, advice.

Never fear, as trainers we get a lot of that in the gym, and we know how you feel. The formula for losing weight is surprisingly simple: burn more calories than you take in, you lose weight. Eat fewer calories, stay active, and burn stored fat for energy – simple, right?

And yet, the myths just keep on coming. So, to ease your mind, quiet the water cooler chorus, and keep you on track, let's address some of the "facts" we both know you've probably already heard…

SKINNYCHEATS
The Trainers Secrets

Cutting carbohydrates will help you lose weight.

Fact: The short-term effects of cutting carbs include fatigue, constipation, irritability, and bingeing. Long-term effects (months and years) can include an elevated risk of heart disease and colon cancer.

Eating fattening foods causes rapid weight gain.

Fact: It takes 3,500 extra calories to gain one pound. Two ounces of chocolate or a small bag of chips is not going to cause you to gain five pounds overnight. Remember that it's not what you eat at one meal that causes weight gain: It's the extra calories you eat and store, meal after meal.

Know that if you get on the scale in the evening, you have not only your body weight on that scale, you've got fluid and food weight, as well.

Low-fat foods will help you drop the extra weight.

Fact: The bottom line on this one is that low-fat never means no-fat. Fat-free is not calorie-free. In order to reduce the calories and fat, manufacturers add extra sugars and thickeners to make the foods look and taste like the versions we're used to, and the result can be almost as high in fat and calories as the originals.

Diets don't work for permanent weight loss.

Fact: Diets alone are not the best way to lose keep weight off permanently. Most people quickly get tired of them and regain any lost weight. For permanent weight loss, you are going to have to change your eating lifestyle. You will absolutely have to exercise and watch the addition of fats, alcohol and sugar to your regular eating.

Tip: Research suggests that losing ½ to 2 pounds a week by making healthy food choices, eating moderate portions, and building physical activity into your daily life is the best way to lose weight and keep it off. By adopting healthy eating and physical activity habits, you may also lower your risk for developing:

- type 2 diabetes
- heart disease
- high blood pressure

High Protein / Low Carb Diets are a healthy way to lose weight and keep it off.

Fact: The long-term health effects of a high-protein/low-carbohydrate diet are unknown. But getting most of your daily calories from high-protein foods like meat, eggs, and cheese is not a long-term, balanced eating plan. You may be eating too few fruits, vegetables, and whole grains, which may lead to constipation due to lack of dietary fiber. Following a high-protein/low-carbohydrate diet may also make you feel:

- nauseous
- tired
- weak

Tip: High-protein/low-carbohydrate diets are often low in calories because food choices are limited, so they may cause short-term weight loss. A reduced-calorie eating plan that includes recommended amounts of carbohydrate, protein, and fat will also allow you to lose weight. You may also find it easier to stick with a diet or eating plan that includes a greater variety of foods.

Starches are fattening and should be limited when trying to lose weight.

Fact: Many foods high in starch, are low in fat and calories such as:

- bread
- rice
- pasta
- cereals
- beans
- fruits
- some vegetables (like potatoes and yams)

They become high in fat and calories when eaten in large portions or when covered with high-fat toppings like butter, sour cream, or mayonnaise.

Tip: The US Dietary Guidelines for Americans recommend eating 6 to 11 servings a day, depending on your calorie needs, from the bread, cereal, rice, and pasta group – even when trying to lose weight. Pay attention to your serving sizes and try to avoid high-fat toppings when choosing whole grains, like:

- whole wheat bread
- brown rice
- oatmeal
- bran cereal

"I can lose weight while eating whatever I want."

SKINNYCHEATS
The Trainers Secrets

Fact: To lose weight, you need to use more calories than you eat. It is possible to eat any kind of food you want and lose weight. You need to limit the number of calories you eat every day and increase your daily physical activity. Portion control is also extremely important.

Tip: When trying to lose weight, you can still eat your favorite foods, as long as you pay attention to the portion sizes, and the total number of calories consumed.

Low fat or nonfat means no calories.

Fact: A low-fat or nonfat food is often lower in calories than the same size portion of the full-fat product, but many processed low-fat or nonfat foods have just as many (and sometimes more) calories as the full-fat version of the same food because of added sugar, flour, or starch thickeners to improve flavor and texture after fat is removed.

Tip: Read the Nutrition Facts Label on a food package to find out how many calories are in a serving. Check the serving size too -- it may be less than you expect.

Fast foods are always an unhealthy choice and will always lead to weight gain.

Fact: Fast foods can be part of a healthy weight loss program, if you're smart about portion sizes, and watching fat and sugars in your choices.

Tip: Avoid supersizing your meals, or split the entrée and desert with a friend. Make fast friends with water – it fills you up, is good for you, and aids in digestion. Choose salads with vinaigrette dressings instead of the high fat creamy varieties. Go for the grilled foods, instead of the fried – frying can multiply the calorie count of your otherwise innocent chicken breast by four (4!). Fried foods, like French fries and fried chicken, are high in fat and calories, so if you have to have them, order a small portion, or split an order with a friend. Also, use only small amounts of high-fat, high-calorie toppings, like:

- regular mayonnaise
- salad dressings
- bacon
- cheese

Skipping meals is a good way to lose weight.

Fact: Studies show that people who skip breakfast and eat fewer times during the day tend to be heavier than people who eat a healthy breakfast and eat four or five times a day. This may be because people who skip meals tend to feel hungrier later on, and eat more than they normally would.

Tip: Eat small meals throughout the day that include a variety of healthy, low-fat, low-calorie foods.

Eating after 8pm causes weight gain.

Fact: It does not matter what time of day you eat. It is what and how much you eat, and how much physical activity you do during the whole day that determines whether you gain, lose, or maintain your weight. No matter what time you eat, your body will store extra calories as fat.

Tip: If you want to eat late, think about how many calories you have eaten that day. And try to avoid snacking in front of the TV -- it may be easier to overeat when you are distracted by the television.

Lifting weights while dieting will lock in the fat and "bulk you up".

Fact: Lifting weights or doing strengthening activities on a regular basis can actually help you maintain or lose weight. Strength training helps to build muscle. Muscle, even at rest, burns calories continuously. Doing strengthening activities will not "bulk you up." Only intense strength training, combined with a specific diet and genetic background, will build very large muscles.

Tip: In addition to doing at least 30 minutes of moderate-intensity physical activity (like walking 2 miles in 30 minutes) on most days of the week, try to do strengthening activities 2 to 3 days a week. You can:

- lift weights
- use resistance bands
- do push-ups or sit-ups

Nuts are fattening and eating them will prevent your losing weight.

Fact: In small amounts, nuts can be part of a healthy weight loss program. While nuts are high in calories and fat, most nuts contain healthy fats that do not clog arteries.

Tip: Nuts are also good sources of protein, dietary fiber, and minerals including magnesium and copper. Enjoy small portions of nuts. One-third cup of mixed nuts has about 270 calories.

Eating red meat makes it hard to lose weight.

Fact: Eating lean meat in small amounts can be part of a healthy weight-loss plan. Red meat, pork, chicken, and fish all contain some cholesterol and saturated fat (the least healthy kind of fat). They also contain healthy nutrients like protein, iron, and zinc.

• **Tip:** Choose cuts of meat that are lower in fat and trim all visible fat. Also, pay attention to portion size. One serving is 2 to 3 ounces of cooked meat.

Dairy products are fattening and lead to high levels of blood fat (cholesterol).

Fact: Low-fat and nonfat milk, yogurt, and cheese are just as nutritious as whole milk dairy products, but they are lower in fat and calories.

• **Tip:** The Dietary Guidelines for Americans recommend that people aged 9 to 18 and over age 50 have three servings of milk, yogurt, and cheese a day. Adults aged 19 to 49 need two servings a day, even when trying to lose weight. A serving is equal to 1 cup of milk or yogurt, 1½ ounces of natural cheese such as cheddar, or 2 ounces of processed cheese such as American.

If you cannot digest the sugar found in dairy products (lactose), choose low-lactose or lactose-free dairy products, or other foods and beverages that offer calcium and vitamin D, including:

Calcium: fortified fruit juice, soy-based beverage, or tofu made with calcium sulfate; canned salmon; dark leafy greens like collards or kale.

Vitamin D: fortified fruit juice, soy-based beverage, or cereal (getting some sunlight on your skin also gives you a small amount of vitamin D.

A vegetarian diet is a "sure fire" way to lose weight.

Fact: Research shows that people who follow a vegetarian eating plan, tend to eat fewer calories and less fat than non-vegetarians. They also tend to have lower body weights relative to their heights than non-vegetarians. Choosing a vegetarian eating plan with a low fat content may be helpful for weight loss, but vegetarians still have to make healthy choices and be wary of eating large amounts of high-fat, high-calorie foods, or choosing foods with little or no nutritional value.

Tip: Choose a vegetarian eating plan that is low in fat and provides all of the nutrients your body needs. Food and beverage sources of nutrients that may be lacking in a vegetarian diet include:

Iron: cashews, spinach, lentils, garbanzo beans, fortified bread or cereal

Calcium: dairy products, fortified soy-based beverages or fruit juices, tofu made with calcium sulfate, collard greens, kale, broccoli

Vitamin D: fortified foods and beverages including milk, soy-based beverages, fruit juices, or cereal

Vitamin B12: eggs, dairy products, fortified cereal or soy-based beverages, tempeh, and miso

Zinc: whole grains, nuts, tofu, leafy vegetables like spinach, cabbage, and lettuce.

Protein: eggs, dairy products, beans, peas, nuts, seeds, tofu, tempeh, soy-based burgers.

Cheating on a diet is a sure way to stay fat.

Fact: You can gain weight eating anything. The important thing to remember is that it's not what you eat one time – it's what you eat meal, after meal. That means that it's not the "cheat" that counts. It's the habits you form for your present AND your future.

Tip: Think about your "cheat" and how or what you're willing to do about it. It takes 3,500 calories to build a pound of fat. Are you willing to put in a few more minutes of exercise to burn those calories off (think an extra 500 calories every day. 500 calories x 7 days = 3,500 calories).

PART III
THE DIETS

At the beginning of each diet, look for this table and learn:

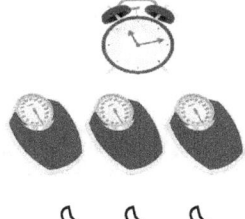

How long our trainers tried each plan.

How much weight they lost.

What they thought of the plan.

Recipes for all of the following food plans are included in the Appendix of this book. Any dish followed by a pair of asterisks (**) is included – we hope you'll enjoy them…

We did!

The Apple Cider Vinegar Diet

Two trainers gave this plan 14 days. Results began to register AFTER day 4 for both of them.

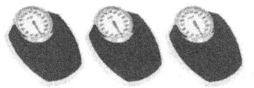

Our scale showed a total of 11 and 13 pounds dropped – nearly a pound per day.

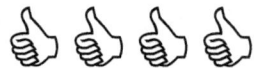

The trainers agreed that Apple Cider Vinegar tastes better than you might expect.

The diet is divided into seven days, and can be repeated indefinitely, if you choose – though more than 14 consecutive days has been found to reduce effectiveness of this plan for most people.

One of the good things about this plan is that you don't have to do the days in any specific order. Day 1 doesn't have to automatically follow Day 2. You can rotate the days to suit yourself – the only thing to remember is that you must, never combine meals from different days. Doing so will change the calorie and chemical balance of the diet and drastically reduce your results.

Day 4 let's you have **a** (read that as ONE!) treat. You are not allowed to do this more than once a week, and ONLY with the Day 4 dinner combination.

Refer to the recommended serving sizes found in the Appendix. When using the suggested recipes, also found in the Appendix (**), try to stick to them as closely as possible. If you decide to amend this program for a longer period of use, experiment with other ingredients (especially sugar and fats) very slowly.

Day 1

Waking-up: 8 ounces water and 1 teaspoon of Apple Cider Vinegar

Breakfast: ½ grapefruit

Oatmeal

Coffee / tea

8 ounces water and 1 teaspoon of Apple Cider Vinegar

Mid morning: Fruit and ½ glass of skim milk.

Lunch: Garden salad with egg and dressing

Mid afternoon: Fruit and ½ glass of skim milk.

Dinner: 8 ounces water and 1 teaspoon of Apple Cider

Vinegar

Grilled, steamed, or poached fish

Steamed vegetables

Green salad

Tea

Day 2

Waking-up: 8 ounces water and 1 teaspoon of Apple Cider Vinegar

Breakfast: ½ papaya

Oatmeal

Coffee or tea

8 ounces water and 1 teaspoon of Apple Cider Vinegar

Mid morning: Slice of whole wheat or multi-grain toast with 1 teaspoon of honey

Lunch: Mixed green salad and grilled or baked fish may be added

Mid afternoon: ½ cup yogurt

1 hour before Dinner: drink 8 ounces water and 1 teaspoon of Apple Cider Vinegar

Dinner: Chicken

Steamed vegetables or Broccoli soup **

Coffee or tea

Day 3

Waking-up: 8 ounces water and 1 teaspoon of Apple Cider Vinegar

Breakfast: ½ cantaloupe

Oatmeal

Coffee or tea

8 ounces water and 1 teaspoon of Apple Cider Vinegar

Mid morning: Apple

Lunch: Half an avocado with salt, pepper and a couple of drops of lemon juice or apple cider vinegar, and 1 slice of bread

or

Some of the Broccoli soup ** from the night before

Mid afternoon: Banana

1 hour before Dinner: drink 8 ounces water and 1 teaspoon of Apple Cider Vinegar

Dinner: Chicken

Health salad **

Fresh fruit salad **

Coffee or tea

Day 4

Waking-up: 8 ounces water and 1 teaspoon of Apple Cider Vinegar

Breakfast: ½ grapefruit

Oatmeal

Coffee or tea

8 ounces water and 1 teaspoon of Apple Cider Vinegar

Mid morning: ½ cup yogurt

Lunch: Fresh fruit salad **

8 ounces water and 1 teaspoon of Apple Cider Vinegar

Afternoon: Toast with honey

1 hour before Dinner: drink 8 ounces water and 1 teaspoon of Apple Cider Vinegar

Dinner: Pasta with Tomato, Basil, and Ricotta **

Green salad

Tea

Choose a treat! Watch portion sizes and choose something you truly want to enjoy eating. Cheesecake, ice cream, a glass of wine... the choice is yours.

Day 5

Waking-up: <u>8 ounces water and 1 teaspoon of Apple Cider Vinegar</u>

Breakfast: ½ grapefruit

Oatmeal

Coffee / tea

8 ounces water and 1 teaspoon of Apple Cider Vinegar

Mid morning: Fruit

Lunch: Pasta with Tomato, Basil, and Ricotta **

or

Chicken breast sandwich with tomato and cucumber slices.

Mid Afternoon: Apple

1 hour before Dinner: drink 8 ounces water and 1 teaspoon of Apple Cider Vinegar

Dinner: Baked potato with sour cream and fresh chives

Health salad **

Coffee / Tea

Day 6

Waking-up: 8 ounces water and 1 teaspoon of Apple Cider Vinegar

Breakfast: ½ grapefruit

Oatmeal

Coffee / tea

8 ounces water and 1 teaspoon of Apple Cider Vinegar

Mid morning: Fresh fruit

Lunch: Health salad **

8 ounces water and 1 teaspoon of Apple Cider Vinegar

Mid afternoon: Open-faced sandwich (made with one slice of bread your choice of chicken, cheese, or tuna, sliced tomato, and field greens)

1 hour before Dinner: drink 8 ounces water and 1 teaspoon of Apple Cider Vinegar

Dinner: 3 – 6 ounces lean beef or pork, grilled

Health salad **

Tea or Coffee

Day 7

Waking-up: 8 ounces water and 1 teaspoon of Apple Cider Vinegar

Breakfast: ½ grapefruit

Oatmeal

Coffee or tea

8 ounces water and 1 teaspoon of Apple Cider Vinegar

Mid morning: ½ cucumber and tomato

Lunch: Tuna salad **

Mid afternoon: Fruit

1 hour before Dinner: drink 8 ounces water and 1 teaspoon of Apple Cider Vinegar

Dinner: Broccoli soup **

3 – 6 ounces fish, beef, pork or chicken, grilled or broiled

Health salad **

Tea or Coffee

The Cabbage Soup Diet

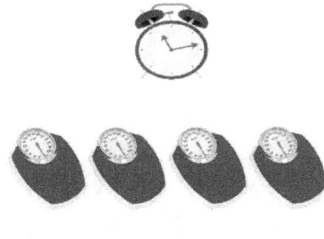

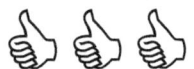

The trainer gave this plan 14 days. Results began to register AFTER day 2.

16 pounds dropped – nearly a pound per day.

The trainer ate an ocean of Cabbage Soup and says that the soup is tasty, and you are NEVER hungry on this plan, but she got tired of making AND eating the soup.

The cabbage soup can be eaten at any time you feel hungry during the day, and you can eat as much as you wish as often as you like.

Soup:

6 Large Green Onions

SKINNYCHEATS
The Trainers Secrets

2 Green Peppers

1-2 Cans Diced Tomatoes

1 Bunch Celery

1 Package Lipton Onion Soup Mix

1-2 Cubes of Bouillon (if desired)

1 head cabbage

Cut vegetables into small pieces and cover with water. (V-8 juice and water can be used). Boil fast for 10 minutes. Reduce to simmer and continue cooking until vegetables are tender. Season to taste with salt, pepper, parsley, etc. EAT AS MUCH AS YOU WANT WHENEVER YOU WANT ANY TIME OF THE DAY.

Diet Plan:

Day One:

Fruit: Eat all of the fruit you want (EXCEPT BANANAS). Eat only your soup and the fruit for the first day. For drinks, select unsweetened teas, cranberry juice and water.

Day Two:

Vegetables: Eat until you are stuffed with fresh, raw or cooked vegetables of your choice. Try to eat leafy green vegetables and stay away from dry beans, peas and corn. Eat all the vegetables you want along with your soup. At dinner, reward yourself with a big baked potato with butter. Do not eat fruit today.

Day Three:

Mix Days One and Two: Eat all the soup, fruits and vegetables you want. NO BAKED POTATO.

Day Four:

Bananas and Skim Milk: Eat as many as eight bananas and drink as many glasses of skim milk as you would like on this day, along with your soup. This day is supposed to lessen your desire for sweets.

Day Five:

Beef And Tomatoes: Ten to twenty ounces of beef and up to six fresh tomatoes. Drink at least 6 to 8 glasses of water this day to wash the uric acid from your body. Eat your soup at least once this day. You may eat broiled or skinless baked chicken instead of beef.

Day Six:

Beef and Vegetables – you may substitute fish, if you prefer. Eat to beef and vegetables to your heart's content on this day. You can even have 2 or 3 steaks if you like, with leafy green vegetables. NO BAKED POTATO. Eat your soup at least once.

Day Seven:

Brown rice, unsweetened fruit juices and vegetables: Again stuff yourself, and be sure to eat your soup at least once this day.

Soup Nutrition Facts

Serving Size 42 g

Amount Per Serving

Calories

10

Calories from Fat

1

% Daily Value*

Total Fat

0.1g

0%

Cholesterol

0mg

0%

Sodium

6mg

0%

Total Carbohydrates

2.4g

1%

Dietary Fiber

0.9g

4%

Sugars

1.3g

Protein

0.6g

| Vitamin A 3% | • | Vitamin C 29% |
| Calcium 2% | • | Iron 2% |

Nutrition Grade A

* Based on a 2000 calorie diet

The Chicken Soup Diet

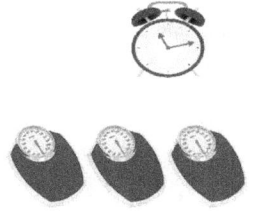

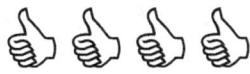

The trainers gave this plan 14 days. Results began to register AFTER day 3.

15 and 17 pounds dropped by the trainers– a little more than a pound per day.

The trainers swear they've eaten an ocean of this tasty Chicken Soup. The soup is delicious and filling – not as boring as the Cabbage Soup. They both hated the breakfast choices, though they promise that you won't be hungry on this plan. And because the soup is so satisfying, it wasn't difficult to go back to a wholesome way of eating.

SKINNYCHEATS
The Trainers Secrets

The Chicken Soup Diet is a very simple plan. You have one of the recommended breakfasts each day (see breakfast choices listed below) and eat as much chicken soup as you want during the day.

Soup:

2 Tablespoons olive or canola oil

4 parsnips cut into ½-inch pieces (this is about 1 pound. of parsnips)

4 ribs celery sliced

1 turnip cut into ½-inch pieces (3/4 of a pound)

1 jalapeno pepper, seeded and chopped

1 Tablespoon chopped garlic

2 teaspoons salt

½ teaspoon cayenne pepper

16 cups reduced fat, low sodium, chicken broth,

7 cans (5 ounces each) of chicken, or 5 cups (1-½ lbs) fresh chicken (cooked)

1 bag (16 ounces) frozen carrots

1 box (10 ounces) frozen broccoli florets

1 box (10 ounces) frozen chopped collard greens

1-½ cups frozen chopped onions

¼ cup lemon juice

¼ cup chopped fresh dill or 1 tbs dried dill.

Cooking Instructions:

SKINNYCHEATS
The Trainers Secrets

In a large pot, heat the oil over medium heat. Add parsnips, celery, turnip, jalapeno pepper, garlic, salt and cayenne pepper. Cook vegetables until they are crisp-tender – about 15 minutes. Add the broth, chicken, carrots, broccoli, collard greens, onions, lemon juice and dill. Bring to a boil, reduce heat and simmer for 5 minutes. Make 26 cups of soup.

Breakfast Choices:

On the Chicken Soup Diet you are allowed one breakfast choice each day. You can try a different breakfast every day, or stick with the ones that suit you best. Since there are only 5 different ones to choose from, for the last two days of the diet, repeat the ones you liked the best.

Breakfast 1: 1 cup vanilla nonfat yogurt combined with ½ cup chopped fruit salad and sprinkled with wheat germ.

Breakfast 2: 1 cup ricotta cheese combined with ½ teaspoon of sugar and a dash of cinnamon.

2 pieces while-grain bread, toasted

3 dried figs

Breakfast 3: 1-½ cups Total cereal

½ cup nonfat milk

½ cup calcium enriched orange juice

Breakfast 4: ½ cup prune juice

1 small whole-wheat bagel

1 ounce of fat-free cheddar cheese

Breakfast 5: 1-½ cups cooked Wheatena Cereal

½ cup nonfat milk

Remember, that you should have one of these breakfasts every day, and then eat **as much of the chicken soup as you want during the day**.

Soup Nutrition Facts

Serving Size 1 cup

Amount Per Serving

Calories
12
Calories from Fat
10

% Daily Value*

Total Fat
1.1g
2%

Cholesterol
0mg
0%

Sodium
180mg
7%

Total Carbohydrates
0.6g
0%

Protein
0.1g

| Vitamin A 1% | • | Vitamin C 3% |
| Calcium 1% | • | Iron 1% |

Nutrition Grade B
* Based on a 2000 calorie diet

The Grapefruit Diet

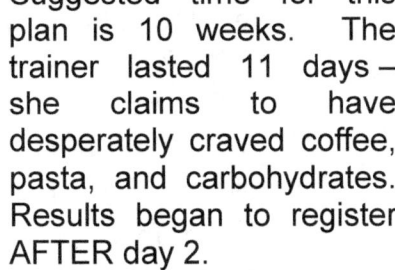

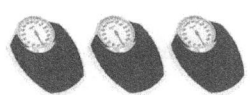

Suggested time for this plan is 10 weeks. The trainer lasted 11 days – she claims to have desperately craved coffee, pasta, and carbohydrates. Results began to register AFTER day 2.

9 pounds dropped – nearly a pound per day.

The menu is boring, but filling, and you are advised to eat until full, but there are so many rules!

The Rules:

- You must drink eight 8 ounces glasses of water daily (64 ounces total per day – minimum).

SKINNYCHEATS
The Trainers Secrets

- You must eat the minimum amount of food listed at each meal.

- You cannot eliminate anything from the diet. Especially the bacon at breakfast and the salads. These combinations of food will burn the fat.

- Omitting any part or combination of foods listed for this plan will cause the whole plan not to work.

- The grapefruit juice is important because it acts as a catalyst to the fat burning process. Don't add or reduce the amount of juice.

- Cut down on coffee. The caffeine content hinders the calorie burning process. Try to limit yourself to 1 cup of black coffee at meal time, if you REALLY have to have it.

- Don't eat between meals. If you eat the suggested foods, you should never be hungry.

- You can fry food in butter and use butter generously on vegetables.

- Do not eat desserts, breads, white vegetables, or sweet potatoes. The sugar content will interfere with calorie burn.

- Stay on the diet 12 days, then stop the diet for 2 days and repeat.

Permitted Foods

Bell Peppers	Green Beans	Pickles (Dill or Bread and Butter)
Broccoli	Green Onions	
Cabbage	Green Vegetables	Radishes
Carrots	Hot Dogs	Red Onions
		Garden Salad

SKINNYCHEATS
The Trainers Secrets

Cheese (any kind)

Chili without Beans

Cole Slaw

Cucumbers

Leaf Spinach

Lettuce

Mayonnaise

Nuts (Dried, 1 teaspoon.)

Dressings

Tomatoes

Excluded Foods

Celery

Cereal

Corn

Corn Chips

Dried Beans or Peas

Fruit Jellies or Jams

Low/Reduced-fat Salad Dressings

Pasta

Peas

Peanut Butter

Potato Chips

Potatoes

Pretzels

Starchy Vegetables

Sweet Pickles

White Onions

Diet Plan:

Breakfast: 8 ounces juice (unsweetened)

2 eggs any style

2 slices of bacon

Lunch: 8 ounces juice (unsweetened)

Salad with any dressing

Meat, any style and any amount

Dinner: 8 ounces juice (unsweetened)

Salad with any dressing, OR a red or green vegetable cooked in butter or spices.

Meat or Fish, any style, cooked any way.

Coffee or Tea (1 cup)

Bedtime Snack Choices:

8 ounces of tomato juice, or 8 ounces of skim milk.

The Ice Cream Diet

Three trainers gave this plan the full 3 days, then repeated it the following weekend, and again on the following weekend. Results began to register on day 2 for all 3 trainers.

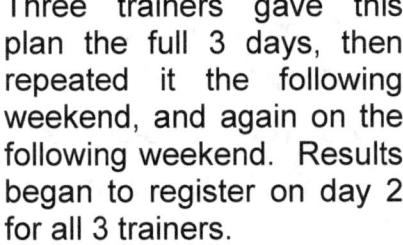

This plan demonstrates the Law of Diminishing Returns: One tester lost 9 pounds in week 1, then 6 pounds in week 2, and 4 pounds in week 3. Another lost 6 pounds each time, and the third lost 10 pounds the first time, nothing week 2, and 5 in week 3.

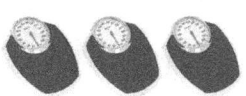

The food combinations are anything but typical. The good thing is that though the results did vary, the unusual combinations did drop weight.

Got a short attention span or need to have immediate results? This may be the plan for you. You have to go on the diet for only three days – and then revert to normal, sensible eating for four days, before tackling it again.

Our dietitian friends say they have no idea where the diet originated, but they agree that this "miracle diet" works on the chemical break-down of certain foods in the body. It delivers an average of 1,000 calories per day – and lets you eat ice cream.

Remember to follow these guidelines:

- Consult your doctor before starting the diet.
- Do not skip meals.
- Drink 8 – 12 8-ounce glasses of water daily.
- Do not add fats when preparing food.
- This diet should be used for three days – followed by four days of normal eating.

Day One

Breakfast: ½ grapefruit

1 slice toast

2 Tablespoons peanut butter

Lunch: ½ cup plain tuna
1 slice toast
black coffee or tea

Dinner: 4 – 6 ounces of any meat
1 cup of string beans
1 cup of beets
1 small apple
1 cup vanilla ice cream

Day 2

Breakfast: 1 egg
½ banana
1 slice toast
black coffee or tea

Lunch: 1 cup cottage cheese
6 saltine crackers

Dinner: 2 hot dogs
1 cup broccoli
½ cup carrots
½ banana
½ cup vanilla ice cream

Day 3

Breakfast: 5 saltine crackers
1 slice cheddar cheese
1 small apple
black coffee or tea

Lunch: 1 hard boiled egg
1 slice toast

Dinner: 1 cup tuna, plain

1 cup of beets

1 cup of cauliflower

½ cantaloupe

½ cup vanilla ice cream

Important: do not vary any of the above foods, and YES, Vanilla ice cream is an important part of this diet plan.

The Lemonade Diet

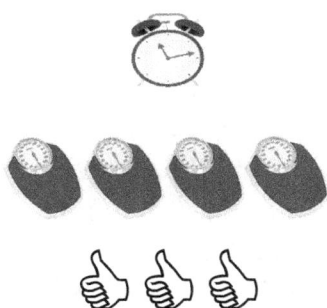

Our trainer gave this plan 14 days. Results began to register AFTER day 4.

18 pounds dropped – more than a pound per day.

The trainer's biggest complaint: She missed CHEWING! It was hard to stick with this one for more than 3 or 4 days.

Our version of this diet is one used by several successful actresses and "top" models who are rumored to swear by this plan. All of the directions we were given for this plan indicate that it should be followed for a minimum of 10 days. Our dietician friends do not recommend this plan for Diabetics.

To make the Lemonade, combine:

2 Tablespoon lemon or lime juice (approx. ½ lemon)

2 Tablespoon genuine maple syrup (not maple flavored sugar syrup)

1/10 teaspoon cayenne pepper (red pepper) or to taste

8 ounces water, medium hot (spring or purified water)

Combine the juice, maple syrup, and cayenne pepper in a 10 ounce glass and fill with water. Use fresh lemons or limes only.

Blend a part of the lemon skin and pulp with the lemonade in a blender for further cleansing and laxative effect.

Mint tea may be used occasionally during this diet as a pleasant change and to assist in the cleansing. Its chlorophyll helps as a purifier, neutralizing many mouth and body odors that are released during the cleansing period.

Drink 6 - 12 glasses of the lemonade daily. If you find that you are hungry during the day, have another glass of lemonade. No other foods will be eaten during the full period of this diet.

Never vary the amount of lemon juice per glass. About six glasses of lemonade a day is enough for those wishing to reduce. You will also need to drink 8 – 12 glasses of water daily.

Coming off the lemonade diet properly is important – please follow the directions very carefully.

FIRST and SECOND DAY AFTER DIET: Several 8 ounces glasses of fresh orange juice as desired during the day. The orange juice prepares the digestive system to properly digest and assimilate regular food. Drink it slowly. If there has been any digestive difficulty prior to or during the change over, extra water may be taken with the orange juice.

THIRD DAY: Orange juice in the morning. Raw fruit for lunch. Fruit or raw vegetable salad at night.

You are now ready to add more kinds of food, but it has to be added gradually:

FIRST DAY: Several 8 ounces glasses of fresh orange juice as desired during the day. Drink it slowly.

SECOND DAY: Drink several 8 ounces glasses of orange juice during the day - with extra water, if needed. Some time during the afternoon prepare Amazing Vegetable Soup**.

Have this soup for the evening meal using the broth mostly, although some of the vegetables may be eaten. Rye wafers may be eaten sparingly with the soup, but no bread or crackers.

THIRD DAY: Drink orange juice in the morning. Enjoy your soup at lunchtime. For the evening meal eat whatever is desired in the form of vegetables, salads, or fruit. No meat, fish, or eggs; no bread, pastries, tea, coffee, or milk.

FOURTH DAY: Normal eating may be resumed.

Lemonade Nutrition Facts
Serving Size 253 g

Amount Per Serving

Calories
8

Calories from Fat
1

% Daily Value*

Total Fat
0.1g
0%

Cholesterol
0mg
0%

Sodium
5mg
0%

Total Carbohydrates
2.5g
1%

Dietary Fiber
0.7g
3%

Sugars
0.7g

Protein
0.3g

| Vitamin A 0% | • | Vitamin C 23% |
| Calcium 1% | • | Iron 1% |

Nutrition Grade A
* Based on a 2000 calorie diet

The Love It and Lose It Diet

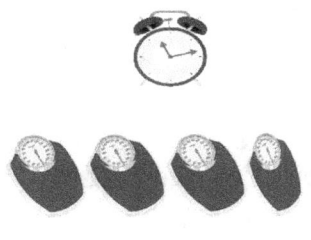

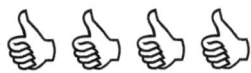

Our trainer gave this plan 21 days. Results began to register AFTER day 5.

9 pounds dropped – not what the trainer was hoping for, but something she could live with.

The recipes are tasty, and when we did a skinfold (caliper) test for body fat, our trainer found a drop of 4%.

This is the most "traditional" eating plan that you will find in this book. It is not the fastest, but it is the one that will lead you to longer term results and good eating habits.

It comes to us, courtesy of a sister-trainer from London. She swears by it and always looks amazing (she tells us) as a result of this plan. Because she's mostly used this plan in England, we had to make some food substitutions, but she's tried this Americanized version, and gives us a BIG thumbs up!

Like many of the other plans included in this book, this one has rules that dictate serving portion sizes, type and number of drinks, low and (relatively) calorie free foods, etc. So, to get you started, here are rules to remember:

- Most portion sizes are given but some are a little bit vague: a handful here and a portion there. These are mostly used for fruits and vegetables where portion size isn't really too important. A fruit portion would be a medium-sized piece of fruit such as an apple, pear or orange, a small banana, two small fruit such as plums or mandarins, a big slice of melon, half a mango, a cupful of berries, cherries or grapes.

- You should add enough vegetables to fill you up – half a pepper, plus half an onion, plus five florets of broccoli, and so on. Veggies are filling, have next to no calories and are so good for you – eat lots of them!

- Plan on spending some time in your kitchen. We've included an abundant supply of recipes (see appendix) to help you stay in control of the fat, sugar, and salt included in your foods.

- Its fine to have tea and coffee (with skim milk and sweeteners if you like) on this plan but stop at four or five per day. Limit diet drinks to an absolute max of two per day and try to cut them out completely if you can.

- With water, more is better – drink one to two liters per day, every day.

- Salads and green veggies are free – the more the merrier!

Make smart choices when eating out...

Restaurant portions are often huge, so it's up to you to make the choices that will keep you on the straight and narrow:

- Portion size: Just because you're in a restaurant doesn't mean that you have to eat everything on the menu or everything you're given. Remember the portion sizes on your plan and eat just until you're satisfied. Get an appetizer and share an entrée, or order two appetizers if the restaurant serves giant portions.

- Healthy choices. You know that a side salad with dressing on the side is a healthier choice than an order of fries or the big bag of chips, so be strong and make the right choice.

- Opt for lean protein (chicken or fish over lamb, lean cuts of beef, etc.), healthy cooking methods (grilled instead of fried, stir-fried instead of deep-fried, etc) and beware of dishes with incredible numbers of fat calories (fat-based gravies or alfredo sauces). Try some of the recipes included in the Appendix of this book.

- Don't go out hungry. Have a snack (fresh fruit, raw veggies, etc.) before going out so that you're not starving and tempted to eat everything.

Takeout meals...

Picking up the prepared takeout meal is fun and easy, but every decision counts. Swapping pepperoni for chicken and extra chili isn't going to ruin your day but it could save you hundreds of calories. Remember to watch portion sizes and factor in the calories when considering fried or heavily sauced choices, when you make your selections.

Frozen and Packaged Choices...

The beauty of getting a prepared, frozen or packaged meal from the supermarket is that you can read the labels and make an informed choice. Your best bet is to go for a meal with less than 400 calories per serving. Be sure to compare different meals to get the best deal for your calories, fat and sodium (the lower the better). Portion sizes can also be big, especially if you get the bagged meal-for-one or meals-for-two. Store anything more than a portion for another meal.

Drinks with friends ...

Alcohol is not your friend when it comes to trying to drop the pounds. Not only does it provide whopping hundreds of calories per sip, but it can also give you the munchies. If you're going for a drink, here's the damage:

> 1.5 ounces alcohol (a standard 80 proof shot): 100 calories (before adding a mixer)
>
> 5 ounce glass of wine: 90-140 calories
>
> 1 wine cooler: 160 calories
>
> 12 ounces of beer: 96 - 150 calories

Enough of the rules, and though we don't want you to forget them, here's the diet:

Week 1

Day 1

Breakfast: Two slices of multi-grain bread, toasted, with low fat margarine (or soy margarine) and two teaspoons of fruit jam.

Snack: Carrot Sprout salad

Lunch: Any canned, frozen, or deli ready-to-go soup. Choose a vegetable, lentil, or bean soup – any choice is fine, as long as it isn't creamy. Add as much salad as you like.

Snack: Low fat yogurt

Dinner: Spicy veggie chili **, and salad or green veggies.

Day 2

Breakfast: Combine a small banana, a big handful of strawberries, a 6 ounce cup of low-fat plain, lemon, or vanilla yogurt, and 6 ounces of skim milk in a blender. Blend until smooth and frothy, and enjoy with ½ whole wheat bagel with low fat margarine (or soy margarine)

Snack: Bag of mini-pretzels – We love the ones we found at Whole Foods.

Lunch: Chicken-In-Foil **, with lots of crisp salad, and a fruit portion.

Dinner: Pick up a ready to go meal at the supermarket deli – remember to look for any meal with less than 400 calories (cut it in half if you need to), and add salad or green veggies.

Day 3

Breakfast: Two slices of multi-grain bread, toasted, with two tablespoons of cottage cheese, and a teaspoon of jam, if you like. Add a 6 ounce glass of orange or grapefruit juice.

Lunch: Tuna salad ** with LOTS of mixed salad greens. Have a fruit portion for dessert.

Afternoon snack: A serving of Chocolate Pudding Cake **

Dinner: Pasta with Tomato, Basil, and Ricotta **, small green salad, and a glass of wine

Day 4

Breakfast: Skinny latte **, with 6 ounces plain (lemon or vanilla may be substituted) yogurt, and 2 tablespoons granola.

Snack: Low-fat yogurt and fruit portion

Lunch: Tired of "brown bagging" it? Visit your local deli for an open faced chicken, turkey, or roast beef sandwich on multigrain roll – keep your choice less than 400 calories. Add a fruit portion.

Dinner: Steak Fajita ** and lots of green salad (watch your dressing!)

Day 5

Breakfast: Bowl of Special K with 6 ounces of skim milk and strawberries

Lunch: Have the rest of Tuna salad ** from day three between two slices of multi-grain bread, with salad and a fruit portion

Snack: Small bag of Sun Chips, or other baked chips.

Dinner: Give yourself a treat and order in or enjoy take-out – but don't forget the RULES! Keep your entrée low in fat and try to stay under 400 calories. Go for the veggies and salad, and desert dessert – missing it will help keep your calorie count down.

SKINNYCHEATS
The Trainers Secrets

Day 6

Breakfast: Whole wheat bagel with 1 ounce cheddar cheese.

Lunch: Any canned, frozen, or deli ready-to-go soup. Choose a vegetable, lentil, or bean soup – any choice is fine, as long as it isn't creamy.

Snack: Portion of fruit and 1 ounce of the cheese of your choice.

Dinner: Enjoy dinner at your favorite restaurant, but don't forget the RULES!

Day 7

Brunch: Fruit salad or juice (even a Virgin Bloody Mary would be fine), eggs or fish or other smart choice served up with lots of veggies. You might even want to try an egg white veggie omelet with salsa.

Snack: Introduce yourself to Edamame, a green vegetable more commonly known as a soybean, used for over two thousand years as a major source of protein. Enjoy a cup, lightly salted or sprinkled with a teaspoon of lemon juice, and you may never eat potato chips again!

Dinner: Pork Stir-Fry **, and lots of green veggies or salad (watch the dressing!)

Snack: Portion of fruit

Week 2

Day 1

Breakfast: Pour 4 ounces of orange juice, 4 ounces of apple juice, and a handful of strawberries into a blender. Blend until smooth, and enjoy.

Snack: Skinny latte ** and a Power Bar

Lunch: Salad Nicoise **. Your fruit portion today is an orange.

Dinner: Vegetable Satay **, and lots of green salad.

Day 2

Breakfast: Combine a cup of water, low fat margarine (or soy margarine), ½ cup of oatmeal, two tablespoons of raisins, and a grated apple (keep the skin on). Enjoy with a cup of low-fat yogurt

Lunch: Any canned, frozen, or deli ready-to-go soup. Choose a vegetable, lentil, or bean soup – any choice is fine, as long as it isn't creamy, and add salad.

Snack: Six crackers (we like water biscuits), with 2 tablespoons Low-fat Hummus **

Dinner: Honey Mustard Pork with Sweet Potato **, and lots of green salad.

Day 3

Breakfast: Bowl of Special K with skim milk and strawberries or blueberries.

Snack: Portion of fruit

Lunch: Fill a large wholegrain pita pocket with 2 tablespoons Low-fat Hummus **, a tablespoon of plain yogurt, 1 tablespoon of black olives, cherry tomatoes and lots of green salad. Enjoy 6 ounces of apple, orange, or grapefruit juice.

Dinner: Pick up your meal from the supermarket or deli (aim for 400 calories or less), with extra salad or vegetables. Select a dessert (200 calories or less).

Day 4

Breakfast: In a blender, mix together a medium-sized banana, 6 ounces of low-fat yogurt, 6 ounces of skim milk and either a few drops of vanilla extract or a pinch of cinnamon. Blend until smooth and enjoy.

Snack: A Kellogg's Nutrigrain or Granola bar

Lunch: Open faced chicken, turkey, or roast beef deli sandwich on multigrain roll – keep your choice less than 400 calories. Add a fruit portion. Remember to read the labels to compare calories, fat and sodium. Add a fruit portion and enjoy.

Dinner: Turkey Frittata Florentine ** and lots of salad.

Day 5

Breakfast: Chop an apple, a small banana, a kiwi fruit and four dried apricots. Mix all the fruit together and top with 6 ounces of low-fat yogurt.

Lunch: Select a frozen entrée (Stouffers, Lean Cuisine, etc).

Snack: Select fresh, crisp baby carrots, sliced cucumbers, broccoli florets, or similar veggies, with 1 tablespoon low-fat ranch dressing for dipping.

Dinner: Enjoy your Friday night takeout with glass of wine! Don't forget the rules.

Day 6

Breakfast: French Toast**, 6 ounces of orange juice

Lunch: Choose a prepared meal – go with one like Lean Cuisine®, Weight Watchers®, or South Beach® and add a fruit portion.

Snack: Portion of fruit

Dinner: Pizza-for-one. Read the labels to find the best choice (not pepperoni!), and tons of salad. A beer (ONE!), if you really want it, is allowed.

Day 7

Breakfast: Grill two turkey sausage patties or links and two tomatoes, halved. Serve with a slice of wholegrain toast, and 6 ounces of orange juice

Lunch: Toasted bagel with three tablespoon low-fat cottage cheese mixed with sliced celery and a sliced spring onion. Season with black pepper and any fresh herbs of your choice, and serve with a salad.

Snack: Banana

Dinner: Salmon pasta ** and salad.

Week 3

Day 1

Breakfast: Toasted bagel with two teaspoons high fruit jam and cottage cheese, extra light cream cheese or natural yogurt

Snack: Fruit juice or smoothie (from our list)

Lunch: Take a trip to the salad bar and enjoy a variety of green, yellow, and red vegetables with a wholegrain roll or breadstick. Avoid the cheeses, croutons, fried add-ons, and creamy dressings.

Dinner: Goulash **, and your choice of green and yellow (orange or red) vegetables

Day 2

Breakfast: Bowl of Special K with skim milk and a handful of dried fruit

Lunch: Choose a prepared meal – go with one like Lean Cuisine®, Weight Watchers®, or South Beach® and add a fruit portion.

Snack: Chocolate Pudding Cake**

Dinner: Choose a prepared meal – go with one like Lean Cuisine®, Weight Watchers®, or South Beach®

Day 3

Breakfast: Skinny latte** with a plain croissant or wholegrain muffin. Read the labels – Muffins can have up to 600 calories each, so be careful!

Lunch: Fill a wholegrain pita pocket with ½ cup Tuna Salad **, 2 tablespoons mixed beans or sprouts, diced cucumber, tomato, spring onion, and add a small side salad

Snack: 1-2 ounces of unsalted Trail Mix

Dinner: Ratatouille **, and veggies of your choice (no rice or potatoes).

Day 4

Breakfast: 6 ounces plain yogurt, a cupful of strawberries or raspberries, and a teaspoon of honey or maple syrup

Snack: Cereal bar

Lunch: Choose a prepared meal – go with one like Lean Cuisine®, Weight Watchers®, or South Beach® and add a fruit portion.

Dinner: Chicken salsa with potato wedges **, and lots of salad.

Day 5

SKINNYCHEATS
The Trainers Secrets

Breakfast: Two slices of multi-grain bread, toasted, with reduced-fat olive spread and a teaspoon or two of high fruit jam.

Lunch: Take a trip to the salad bar and enjoy a variety of green, yellow, and red vegetables with a wholegrain roll or breadstick. Avoid the cheeses, croutons, fried add-ons, and creamy dressings.

Snack: Enjoy your edamame.

Dinner: Italian Sausage and Potatoes **

Day 6

Breakfast: 1 cup oatmeal, topped with a splash of skim milk and a tablespoon of apple sauce.

Lunch: Dig into your veggies today. Select 4 (leave out the potatoes and rice!), then add a wholegrain roll, and a fruit portion

Snack: Select fresh, crisp baby carrots, sliced cucumbers, broccoli florets, or similar veggies, with 1 tablespoon low-fat ranch dressing for dipping.

Dinner: Takeout from your supermarket deli – remember the rules – and a glass of wine.

Day 7

Breakfast: 4 ounces of orange juice, 4 ounces of apple juice and a handful of raspberries (frozen are fine) into a blender. Blend until smooth, and enjoy with ½ toasted whole wheat bagel with 1 teaspoon reduced fat margarine

Lunch: Couscous salad **

Snack: 4 ounces of baked chips or low-salt pretzels

Dinner: Aromatic Lamb Chops ** and lots of green veggies.

Week 4

Day 1

Breakfast: Bowl of Kashi cereal with skim milk, and 6 ounces of fruit juice

Snack: Skinny latte **

Lunch: Go out for soup or sandwich (remember the rules), and add a fruit portion

Dinner: Sweet and Sour Chicken **, 1 serving of rice, and lots of green veggies, or salad

Day 2

Breakfast: Bowl of Special K with skim milk and a handful of dried fruit

Lunch: Choose a prepared meal – go with one like Lean Cuisine®, Weight Watchers®, or South Beach® and add a fruit portion.

Snack: 4 Oatmeal Goodies **

Dinner: Salmon with new potatoes ** and double your vegetables.

Day 3

Breakfast: Chop an apple, a small banana, a kiwi fruit and five ready-to-eat apricots, top with 6 ounces of natural yogurt

Snack: Cereal bar or flapjack slice

Lunch: Go out for soup or sandwich (remember the rules), and add a fruit portion.

Dinner: Choose a prepared meal – go with one like Lean Cuisine®, Weight Watchers®, or South Beach®, with extra salad or veggies, and a glass of wine.

Day 4

Breakfast: Bowl of Special K with skim milk and a handful of dried fruit

Lunch: Fill ½ of a wholegrain pita with Tuna Salad ** or 4 ounces sliced chicken breast, and top with LOTS of mixed salad greens. Add a fruit portion.

Snack: 5 dried apricots and 1 ounce cheddar cheese

Dinner: Pork and Pineapple Kabobs **, with salad.

Day 5

Breakfast: Nutrigrain bar, carton of fruit juice

Lunch: Portabello Mushroom Sandwich **

Snack: Serving of applesauce

Dinner: Choose a prepared meal – go with one like Lean Cuisine®, Weight Watchers®, or South Beach®, and add tons of veggies, or a fruit portion.

Day 6

Breakfast: Wholegrain bread roll, two grilled turkey links or patties, grilled tomato and mushrooms

Lunch: Choose a prepared meal – go with one like Lean Cuisine®, Weight Watchers®, or South Beach® and add a fruit portion.

Snack: Kellogg's Nutrigrain or Cereal Bar

Dinner: Quick beef chili **, lots of salad.

Day 7

Brunch: Fruit salad, or juice, an egg white omelet, containing turkey, chicken, or fish, and lots of veggies is a smart choice

Snack: Two celery sticks with two teaspoons of peanut butter, or Low-fat Hummus **

Dinner: Enjoy a serving of French Bread pizza from Weight Watchers®, Lean Cuisine®, etc – read the labels to find the best choice (here's a hint: not pepperoni!), and tons of salad. A glass of wine would be fine.

The New Mayo Clinic Diet

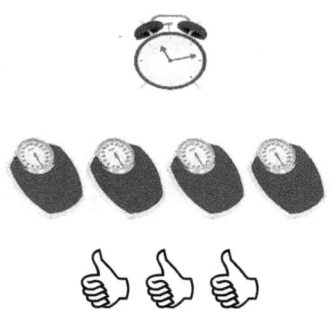

The trainers gave this plan 14 days.   Results began to register AFTER day 3.

19 pounds dropped – more than a pound per day.

Like the Grapefruit Diet, the trainers found that this one worked, but the suggested food combinations were not always to their liking.

Although the New Mayo Clinic Diet is responsible for millions of pounds in weight loss, our research indicates that this diet did not originate at Mayo Clinic, nor is it approved by the Mayo Clinic. The list of rules is long for this one:

- At any meal you may eat until you are full, and cannot eat anymore. You must eat the minimum listed at each meal.

- Do not eliminate anything from the diet. It is the combination of foods that burn the fat.

SKINNYCHEATS
The Trainers Secrets

- Grapefruit is an important part of this diet because it acts as the catalyst for the burning process.

- Don't eat between meals: if you eat the combination of food suggested, you will not get hungry.

- Do not eat desserts, breads and white vegetables or sweet potatoes. You may double or triple helpings of meat, salads or vegetables.

- Stay on this plan a MAXIMUM of 12 days. If you want to repeat it, stay off 2 days, then begin again.

Permitted Foods

Bell Peppers	Green Beans	Pickles (Dill/Bread and Butter)
Broccoli	Green Onions	
Cabbage	Green Vegetables	Radishes
Carrots	Hot Dogs	Red Onions
Cheese (any kind)	Leaf Spinach	Regular Salad Dressings
	Lettuce	
Chili without Beans	Mayonnaise	Tomatoes
Cole Slaw	Nuts (Dried, 1 teaspoon.)	
Cucumbers		

Excluded Foods

Celery	Low/Reduced-fat Salad Dressings	Potatoes
Cereal		Pretzels
Corn	Pasta	Starchy Vegetables
Corn Chips	Peas	
Fruit	Peanut Butter	Sweet Pickles
Jellies or Jams	Potato Chips	White Onions

SKINNYCHEATS
The Trainers Secrets

BREAKFAST:

½ grapefruit or 8 ounces unsweetened juice.

2 eggs any style

2 slices of bacon

black coffee or tea, no sugar

LUNCH:

½ grapefruit or 8 ounces unsweetened juice.

Salad and or raw veggies with dressing

Meat (Cooked any way)

DINNER:

½ grapefruit or 8 ounces unsweetened juice.

Meat (cooked any way)

Vegetables (any green or red, may be cooked in butter or Seasoning or a salad as above)

Black coffee or tea, no sugar

BEDTIME:

8 ounces Tomato juice or skim milk

The Sacred Heart Medical Diet

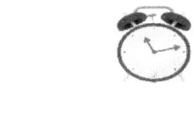

Our trainers gave this plan the full 7 days. Results began to register AFTER day 2.

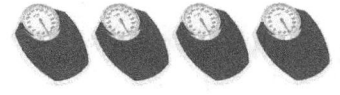

13 pounds dropped by each trainer – nearly 2 pounds per day.

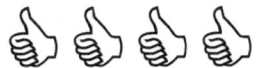

This plan left our trainers feeling even better than expected.

We actually liked this plan a lot, but it does have rules.

- This 7-day eating plan can be used as often as you like. If, by the 7th day, you have lost more than 17 pounds, stay off the diet for two days before resuming the diet again.

- This diet does not lend itself to drinking any alcoholic beverages at any time – alcohol will slow or completely stop your weight loss because of the metabolic effort needed to burn the alcohol.

SKINNYCHEATS
The Trainers Secrets

- After being on the diet for several days, you will find that your elimination habits have changed. If necessary, eat a cup of bran or fiber to increase your bowel movements.

- The basic fat burning soup can be eaten anytime you feel hungry during the seven days. Eat as much as you wish. Remember the more you eat, the more you will lose. You can eat broiled, boiled or baked chicken (Absolutely no skin on the chicken), instead of the beef. If you prefer, you can substitute broiled fish for the beef on only one of the beef days. You need the high protein in the beef for the other days.

Do NOT:	DO:
• Eat bread	• Drink 64 – 128 ounces of water every day
• Drink alcohol	
• Drink carbonated drinks	• Enjoy black coffee, skim milk, or unsweetened fruit drinks, and skim milk,
• Drink diet drinks	
• Eat fried foods	

SOUP:

  1 or 2 cans of stewed tomatoes

  3 plus large green onions

  1 large can of beef broth (no fat)

  1 pkg. Lipton Soup mix (chicken noodle)

  1 bunch of celery

  2 cans green beans

  2 lbs. Carrots

2 Green Peppers

Season with salt, pepper curry, parsley, if desired, or bouillon, hot or Worcestershire sauce. Cut veggies in small to medium pieces. Cover with water. Boil fast for 10 minutes. Reduce to simmer and continue to cook until veggies are tender.

DAY ONE: Any fruit **(except bananas)**. Cantaloupes and watermelon are lower in calories than most other fruits. Eat only soup and fruit today.

DAY TWO: All vegetables. Eat until you are stuffed with fresh raw, cooked or canned veggies. Try to eat green leafy veggies and stay away from dry beans, peas or corn. Eat veggies along with the soup. At dinner time tonight reward yourself with a big baked potato and butter. Don't eat any fruit through today.

DAY THREE: Eat all the soup, fruit and veggies you want. Do not have a baked potato. If you have eaten as above for three days and not cheated, you should find that you have lost 5-7 pounds.

DAY FOUR: Bananas and skim milk: Eat at least 3 bananas and drink as much milk as you can today, along with the soup. Bananas are high in calories and carbohydrates, as is the milk but on this particular day, your body will need the potassium and carbs, proteins, and calcium to lessen the cravings for sweets.

DAY FIVE: Beef and tomatoes: you may have 10 to 20 ounces of beef and a can of tomatoes, or as many as 6 tomatoes on this day. Eat the soup at least once today.

DAY SIX: Beef and veggies, eat to your heart's content of the beef and veggies today. You can even have 2-3 steaks if you like with green leafy veggies but no baked potato. Be sure to eat the soup at least once today.

DAY SEVEN: Brown rice, unsweetened fruit juice and veggies, again, be sure to stuff yourself and eat the soup. You can add cooked veggies to your rice if you wish.

Soup Nutrition Facts

Serving Size 47 g

Amount Per Serving

Calories
17
Calories from Fat
1

% Daily Value*

Total Fat
0.1g
0%

Cholesterol
0mg
0%

Sodium
25mg
1%

Total Carbohydrates
4.0g
1%

Dietary Fiber
1.3g
5%

Sugars
1.9g

Protein
0.5g

Vitamin A 85% • Vitamin C 17%

Calcium 1% • Iron 1%
Nutrition Grade A
* Based on a 2000 calorie diet

The Seven Day "All You Can Eat" Diet

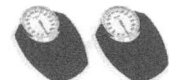

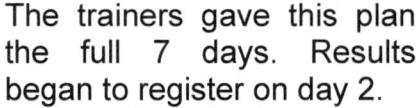

The trainers gave this plan the full 7 days. Results began to register on day 2.

The combined loss for both trainers showed 9 pounds dropped... not nearly enough to justify ever doing this again.

The plan got old. The food was boring and both trainers got diarrhea – really quickly.

This plan is about as simple as they come. The foods are listed for each day. Eat them in the order they are listed. Eat them the way they are listed. Eat until you are full.

MONDAY: All the fruit you want except bananas.

SKINNYCHEATS
The Trainers Secrets

TUESDAY: All the vegetables you want. You may use soy sauce, vinegar, or mustard for extra flavor.

WEDNESDAY: All the fruit & vegetables you want.

THURSDAY: 5 bananas with 5 glasses of milk

FRIDAY: 4 (3-ounce beef/chicken or fish steaks) with fresh vegetables

SATURDAY: 4 (3-ounce beef steaks) with fresh vegetables

SUNDAY: 4 (3-ounce beef steaks) with fresh vegetables

The Trainers Kick Start Diet

Our trainers gave this plan the full 7 days. Results began to register on day 2.

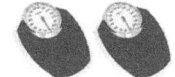

5 and 7 pounds dropped, and our trainers claimed that they were both hungry the whole time.

We don't know the Trainers who came up with this one, but if we did…

Our trainers suggested we save the worst for last…

The Trainers Kickstart diet is more of a starvation plan than a plan for weight loss success. Although it claims to boost metabolism, a starvation diet will accomplish just the opposite by tossing the dieter into metabolic lock-down, slowing body and mind down to a snail's pace to conserve precious calories. All that, and your body will have no idea that you're purposely restricting calorie-intake.

SKINNYCHEATS
The Trainers Secrets

This diet is kind of a mini-version of **The Scarsdale Diet.** The rules of The Trainer's Kickstart Diet Plan:

- Drink a minimum of 4 glasses of water or diet beverage per day.

- Any of the following may be used to your heart's content: salt, pepper, vinegar, lemon, herbs, Worcestershire sauce, soy sauce, mustard and catsup.

Day 1

Breakfast: Coffee or Tea with sugar substitute

Lunch: 2 hard-boiled eggs, 1 cup spinach

Dinner: Lettuce and Celery salad **, 6 ounces grilled or broiled steak

Day 2

Breakfast: Coffee or Tea with sugar substitute, and 6 saltine crackers

Lunch: Lettuce and Celery salad**, 6 ounces grilled or broiled steak

Dinner: 8-10 ounces of lean ham

Day 3

Breakfast: Coffee or Tea with sugar substitute, and 6 saltine crackers

Lunch: 2 hard-boiled eggs, 1 cup of green beans, and 1 cup of tomatoes

Dinner: 8 - 10 ounces of lean ham, 2 cups of green beans, and tomato salad **

SKINNYCHEATS
The Trainers Secrets

Day 4

Breakfast: Coffee or Tea with sugar substitute, and 6 saltine crackers

Lunch: 1 hard-boiled egg, and 1 cup of carrots

Dinner: 1 cup of plain REGULAR yogurt, 1 ounce of Mozzarella cheese, and 1 cup of fruit salad **

Day 5

Breakfast: Coffee or Tea with sugar substitute, 1 raw carrot, the juice from one lemon

Lunch: 4 -6 ounce fried fish fillet, and tomato salad **

Dinner: 4 - 6 ounces grilled or broiled steak, and a green salad

Day 6

Breakfast: Coffee or Tea with sugar substitute

Lunch: 4 - 8 ounces grilled or broiled skinless chicken

Dinner: 2 hard-boiled eggs, and 1 raw carrot

Day 7

Breakfast: Tea with lemon

Lunch: 4 - 8 ounce grilled or broiled steak, 1-½ cups fruit salad **

Dinner: 4 – 6 ounces grilled or broiled lean meat or fish

Part III
WAYS TO "AMP" IT UP

The Herbal Assist

Sometimes, when you're trying to work your way into your best body, you need a little help. And, while we all know that everything natural isn't always in our best interest (anybody know what a "cow pie" is? Eeww!). A weight loss product that claims to be *natural* or *herbal* is not necessarily safe. For example, herbal products containing ephedra have caused serious health problems and even death. Newer products claiming to be ephedra-free are not necessarily danger-free, because they may contain ingredients similar to ephedra.

And while the trainers are not enthused about products like those containing ephedra, we are not doctors. Talk with your health care provider before using any weight loss product. Our list will provide help in making an informed choice. Though the listed herbs are not prescriptions, you still need to confer with your physician – especially if you are taking any medications.

Nobody ever said there was a "magic bullet" for knocking off the pounds, and we certainly don't want you to think that trainers are running around recommending herbs to all their clients. Eating a healthy diet and exercising are still essential if you want to succeed but herbs can make the process of losing weight a bit easier.

There is a sincere argument in favor of herbs that can increase your stamina and help you to get through a workout. If your interest is indeed in herbs, some of the ones you'll want to investigate are:

St. Johns Wort Most often considered an herbal antidepressant, it is also a tonic that strengthens the nervous system. Ensuring a steady supply of the neuro-transmitters needed for proper nerve function. It is the herbal choice if you tend to succumb to overeating under stress.

Cayenne

(Capsicum minima)

This most famous thermogenic herb offers more than just a hot mouth: eaten, it makes you sweat and warms your fingers and toes. It can also offer relief to arthritic joints and bones when blended into an emollient. Red pepper also jump-starts your circulation and gets your blood rushing to pick up your metabolic rate.

Cordyceps

(Cordyceps sinensis)

Cordyceps is an ancient Chinese remedy famous for increasing stamina and well being. Once an extremely rare and costly herb, contemporary production techniques have made this mushroom more affordable. Bodybuilders use it to power up workout sessions and endurance athletes use it to enhance stamina.

Flaxseed

(linum usitatissimum)

Used as a soothing bulking agent, the seed of the flax plant is covered with mucilage, which swells in water, much like the psyllium seed. Used as a laxative, whole seeds go through the body largely undigested and unabsorbed.

Ginger

(Zingiber officinale)

Like cayenne, ginger is a thermogenic herb. It stimulates blood flow and stirs the blood to raise your metabolic rate, and burn calories. It's also said to aid in soothing arthritic joints when used as a tea or compress.

Oat Straw

In the previous century, holistic physicians found this herb helped alcoholics, smokers and heroin addicts to overcome symptoms of withdrawal. If you are having a difficult time with willpower, find some oat straw.

Psyllium

(Plantago psyllium)

The seed of the Indian plantain has an almost pure fiber coating. When exposed to water, it swells to four times its original size. The seed has the added benefit of reducing cholesterol levels while giving you a pleasant, full feeling.

Siberian Gensing

(Eleutherococcu s senticosus)

Long used in Asia, Siberian ginseng increases endurance in humans. Many studies show that this herb increases the capacity to do workouts or other physical activity.

Diuretics

Diuretics are a diverse group of compounds that either stimulate or inhibit various hormones that naturally occur in the body to regulate urine. This can lead to an accelerated metabolism that seems to flush out the fatty deposits that may lodge themselves on cells. The foods that are listed below act as diuretics to help you break down and eliminate fatty deposits from your body.

Remember, the trainers are not doctors. Better still, remember that most trainers are not specifically trained to offer medical advice. That said, we do know that people are inclined to look for the fastest advice they can access, so we're sharing the information we use.

Asparagus   Asparagus contains the chemical asparagine, an alkaloid complex that stimulates the kidneys and improve the circulatory process. Alkaloids directly impact cells and break down fat.

Beets

Beets focus on the liver and kidneys, flushing out floating body fats. Their iron content cleanses the corpuscles, blood cells that can contain fat deposits. Beets also contains chlorine that stimulates the lymphatic system.

Brussels
Sprouts

This vegetable stimulates the glands, the pancreas especially, which releases hormones that have a cleansing effect on the cells. There are also minerals that stimulate the kidneys. Waste is released quicker and it helps to clean out the cells

Cabbage

The sulfur and iodine content of cabbage act to cleanse the mucous membranes of the stomach and intestines. Cabbage is a great food if you should have a potbelly. Cabbage, especially red cabbage is known to be highly effective.

Carrots

The carotene, a form of Vitamin A, in carrots influences a fat flushing reaction in your system. This reaction helps to speed up your metabolism and literally washes fat and waste from your body.

Celery

Raw celery has a high concentration of Calcium in a ready to use form, so when you eat it, the calcium is sent directly to work. This pure form of calcium will ignite your endocrine system. The hormones in your body will break up accumulated fat. Celery also has a high level of magnesium and iron, which will clean out your system.

Cucumber

The high sulfur and silicon content of cucumbers works to stimulate the kidneys and wash uric acid from the body. The process of eliminating uric acid stimulates the removal of fat, on a cellular level.

Garlic

If you read the fat burning foods section you would have seen Garlic on that list, well, it is also a natural diuretic. Garlic oils create a cleansing action in the body. They promote a vigorous peristaltic action, where muscle contracts, loosening fat and breaking it down for elimination from the body.

Horseradish

Horseradish has the amazing effect of dissolving fat in cells, and also has a cleansing effect on the body.

Lettuce

Lettuce contains iron and magnesium. These minerals will enter your spleen, and protect the body from illness. Iron and magnesium will also help the liver to process and eliminate fats and toxins from your blood stream, and increase your metabolism. Select the darker lettuces, coarser lettuces for best results.

Onions	Onions, similar to garlic, have minerals and oils that break down fat deposits and speed up your metabolism.
Radishes	Radishes scrub the mucous membrane of the body because it contains high levels of Iron and Magnesium. These minerals actually help to dissolve fat in the cells.
Tomatoes	Tomatoes have high Vitamin C and Citricmalic-oxalic acids. The acid will accelerate the metabolic process. It also helps the kidneys to release more water and helps to wash away fat.

The natural acids with the enzyme activated minerals prompt the kidneys to filter out large quantities of fatty deposits that are eliminated from your system.

Apple Cider Vinegar	The malic acid in apples creates a fat burning process. The fermentation process causes the vinegar to have constructive acids that join with alkaline elements and minerals in the body, producing a cell scrubbing effect. It also contains high levels of potassium, which has an antiseptic quality that helps to eliminate fat deposits.

Fat Flush Foods

Here is a list of foods that our training experience shows will wake up your metabolism and help you flush fat out of your system.

Apples, Berries, and Fresh Fruits	Apples, berries and most fresh fruits contain pectin in their cell walls. Pectin limits the amount of fat your cells absorb. Once in your system, Pectin has a water binding property. It absorbs watery substances and these watery substances, in turn, bombard the cells and make them release fat deposits.
Citrus Fruits	Citrus fruits like, grapefruit, oranges, tangerines, lemons, and limes contain high concentrations of fat-burning Vitamin C (also called ascorbic acid). Vitamin C can liquefy or dilute fat, making it harder to store and easier to flush out of your system. Vitamin C

works similarly on cholesterol deposits, making it difficult for cholesterol deposits to form in blood vessels.

Garlic

Garlic oil and juice offer significant cellular level protective qualities which help to reduce fatty deposits, when taken orally.

Soybeans

Soybeans contain lecithin, a chemical that has been found to shield cells from accumulating fat. Lecithin is also shown to break down fatty deposits in your body.

Words of Water Wisdom

If you eat right and exercise at the intensity, frequency and duration proper for you, but still can't get rid of a little paunch here and there, you're probably not drinking enough water. Most people are carrying around a few more pounds than they would be if they drank enough water.

Wikipedia defines metabolism as: the complete set of chemical reactions that occur in living cells. These metabolic processes are the basis of life, as they allow cells to maintain their structures, respond to their environments, grow, and reproduce.

There are many forms of metabolism going on in your body right now, but the one you're concerned most about is the metabolism of fat. This is what the liver does when it converts stored fat to energy. The liver has other functions, but fat metabolism is a primary job.

Another of the liver's duties is to pick up the slack for the kidneys, which need water to work properly. If the kidneys are water-deprived, the liver has to do their work along with its own, lowering total productivity and the ability to metabolize fat, setting you up to store fat.

During the first few days of drinking more water than your body is accustomed to, you'll run to the bathroom constantly. What is really happening is that your body is flushing itself of the water it has been storing throughout all those years of being in "survival mode".

As you continue to give your body all the water it could ask for, it gets rid of what it doesn't need. It gets rid of the water it was holding onto in your ankles and your hips and thighs, maybe even around your belly. You are excreting much more than you realize. Trusting that the water will keep coming, your body figures it doesn't need to save these stores anymore and if you keep the water coming, the flushing will eventually cease, allowing you to return to a normal life.

Throughout your life, you've heard that water is good for you, and it's true, water will do wonders for your looks. It flushes out impurities in your skin, leaving you with a clear, glowing complexion. Skin that is becoming saggy, either due to aging or weight loss, plumps up nicely when skin cells are hydrated.

Additionally, water improves muscle tone. Muscles that have all the water they need contract more easily, making your workout more effective and ease post-exercise recovery. And don't get us started on the benefits of water to your ability to improve your sleep – simply because your organs are fueled for better function.

Your basic water formula begins with about 64 ounces of water every day. That's eight 8-ounce glasses of

SKINNYCHEATS
The Trainers Secrets

water. But if you're overweight, you are going to need to add water. You should drink another eight ounces for every 25 pounds of excess weight you carry. You should also increase this if you live in a hot climate or exercise very intensely.

Water consumption should be spread out throughout the day. Try to pick three or four times a day when you can have a big glass of water, and then sip in between. If you feel thirsty, know that you're already becoming dehydrated. The simple solution is to drink when you're not thirsty yet.

Drinking other fluids will certainly help hydrate your body, but the extra calories, sugar, additives and whatever added chemicals a soft drink or juice flavored "ade" contains simply aren't what you need. Instead, try a slice of lemon or lime in the glass, or if you really hate water, try a fruit flavored water. Just make sure to read the labels.

Most experts lean toward cold water, because the stomach absorbs it more quickly. There is also some evidence that cold water might enhance fat burning. On the other hand, warmer water is easier to drink in large quantities, and you might drink more of it without even realizing it.

When you drink all the water you need, you will quickly notice a decrease in appetite. If you're aiming for a leaner, healthier body, especially if you're trying to fast-track weight loss, drinking water is an absolute must.

Fiber and Your Weight

Fiber contains no calories, but it provides the bulk to your diet that gives you the satisfaction of chewing, and the feeling of a full stomach. There are two types of fiber: water-insoluble and water-soluble. Water-insoluble fiber, found in vegetables and whole grain breads and cereals, adds bulk to the diet. Water-soluble fiber is found in fruits, legumes, seeds, and oat products. It exits the stomach more slowly and helps your stomach feel full longer. Foods containing fiber take longer to eat, which means your stomach feels full sooner and you eat less.

Insoluble fiber passes through the body, carrying cancer-causing substances through the digestive tract. Additionally, insoluble fiber helps to prevent or relieve constipation because it exits the body quickly. A diet rich in soluble fiber can help to reduce your risk of stroke, control diabetes, prevent some cancers, and avoid gastrointestinal disorders. Soluble fiber can also help lower your blood cholesterol and lower your risk of cardiovascular disease. Soluble fiber absorbs fluids as it moves through your digestive track. During the process, the fiber dissolves, thickens, and forms a gel. This gel binds itself with acids made from cholesterol from the liver and then carries it out of your body through your waste. Your body is left to pull the cholesterol from your blood stream, reducing your blood cholesterol. As the gel moves slowly through the digestive system, it slows the release of sugar and slows sugar absorption, thereby moderating blood glucose levels.

The National Cancer Institute recommends a daily intake of 20 to 35 grams of fiber. However, most Americans only eat between 10 to 15 grams of fiber per day. Fiber is not the cure all for weight control. However, combined with a nutritious diet, fiber can help you lose weight.

When you're ready to add more fiber to your diet, review the following tips:

- Begin adding fiber slowly to your diet to avoid bloating and gas.

- Eight glasses of water a day is the base recommended amount because fibrous foods draw water from the intestines.

- When possible, consume high-fiber carbohydrates such as an apple instead of the low-fiber carbohydrates found in apple juice.

- Shop for fresh produce (about) twice weekly. Many vegetables lose their nutrients during prolonged refrigeration.

- Avoid wilted, dull or discolored, and bruised fruits and vegetables – they're usually old. By the time the broccoli or spinach has begun to lose its color, it has also lost significant nutritional value.

- Choose small, young, colorful vegetables.

- Select whole grain products (breads, pastas, flours, etc) instead of enriched products for greater nutritional content.

- Visit larger stores or health food stores for whole-grain flours and hard-to-find nuts and seeds.

Controlling your weight is more manageable when you add fiber to a nutritious diet. Fiber will not solve all your weight control problems, but it is a step in the right direction.

APPENDICES

BMI
BODY MASS INDEX

Invented between 1830 and 1850 by the Belgian polymath, Adolphe Quetelet, BMI uses a mathematical formula that takes into account both a person's height and weight. BMI equals a person's weight in kilograms divided by height in meters squared ($BMI=kg/m^2$).

The table below has already done the math and metric conversions. To use the table, find the appropriate height in the left-hand column. Move across the row to the given weight. The number at the top of the column is the BMI for that height and weight.

The BMI is a measure of your weight relative to your height and waist circumference measures abdominal fat. Combining these with information about your additional risk factors yields your risk for developing obesity-associated diseases. The higher your BMI, the greater your chances of developing high blood pressure, having strokes, or heart attacks.

BMI Categories:
- Underweight = <18.5
- Normal weight = 18.5-24.9
- Overweight = 25-29.9
- Obesity = BMI of 30 or greater

BMI Chart

BMI (kg/m²)	20	21	22	23	24	25	26	27	28	29	30	35	40
Height (in.)	Weight (pounds)												
58	96	100	105	110	115	119	124	129	134	138	143	167	191
59	99	104	109	114	119	124	128	133	138	143	148	173	198
60	102	107	112	118	123	128	133	138	143	148	153	179	204
61	106	111	116	122	127	132	137	143	148	153	158	185	211
62	109	115	120	126	131	136	142	147	153	158	164	191	218
63	113	118	124	130	135	141	146	152	158	163	169	197	225
64	116	122	128	134	140	145	151	157	163	169	174	204	232
65	120	126	132	138	144	150	156	162	168	174	180	210	240
66	124	130	136	142	148	155	161	167	173	179	186	216	247
67	127	134	140	146	153	159	166	172	178	185	191	223	255
68	131	138	144	151	158	164	171	177	184	190	197	230	262
69	135	142	149	155	162	169	176	182	189	196	203	236	270
70	139	146	153	160	167	174	181	188	195	202	207	243	278
71	143	150	157	165	172	179	186	193	200	208	215	250	286
72	147	154	162	169	177	184	191	199	206	213	221	258	294
73	151	159	166	174	182	189	197	204	212	219	227	265	302
74	155	163	171	179	186	194	202	210	218	225	233	272	311
75	160	168	176	184	192	200	208	216	224	232	240	279	319
76	164	172	180	189	197	205	213	221	230	238	246	287	328

101

SKINNYCHEATS
The Trainers Secrets

YOUR ACTIVITY LEVEL
USING STEPS/DAY

You already know that if you plan to lose weight, you need to ramp up your activity so that you use (burn off) more calories than you take in (eat), but how do you gauge your current level?

One quick and easy way to get an answer to that question is to snap on a pedometer and start moving. Even an inexpensive pedometer can be used to count the number of steps that you take every day.

In looking at the five levels of activity shown in our chart (based in the Tudor-Locke C. & Bassett, D.R., 2004 study) remember:

- Being sedentary means that you are getting less than 150 minutes of exercise per week – this is considered a health risk.

- Being active is recommended to maintain health.

- Being highly active is recommended when trying to lose weight.

ACTIVITY LEVELS	STEPS / DAY
Sedentary	5,000
Low Active	5,001 – 7,499
Somewhat Active	7,500 – 9,999
Active	10,000 – 11,999
Highly Active	12,000 or more

BODY MONITOR

Accountability is EVERYTHING when you are trying to build new and better habits. Measuring is an easy way to know and understand your body. Be sure to measure yourself at the beginning of your diet, then track your progress over the course of your plan.

Date						
Chest/Bust						
Change						
Waist						
Change						
Abdomen						
Change						
Hip						
Change						
Thigh						
Change						
Weight						
Change						
BMI						

SERVING SIZE
Quick Reference

Food Groups	**One Serving Size Equals...**
Breads, Cereals, Rice, Pasta, and other Grains	• 1 slice bread or 1/2 bagel should equal the size of a hockey puck.
	• 1 serving of cornbread equals a bar of soap.
	• 1 pancake equals a compact disk.
	• 1/2 cup cooked rice equals a paper cupcake wrapper.
	• 1/2 cup pasta equals an ice cream scoop.
	• 1 cup cooked cereal equals ½ of a baseball.
	• 1 cup of cereal (flakes) equals a fist.
Fruits and Vegetables	• One fruit and vegetable serving is equal to one piece the size of a tennis ball or 1/2 cup the size of a light bulb.
	• 1 medium banana equals <u>2</u> servings.
	• ½ cup of raisins equals ½ of a large egg.
	• ½ cup of grapes (about 15) equals the size of a light bulb.
	• ¾ cup of juice equals a

small Styrofoam cup.

- 1 cup of salad greens equals a baseball.
- 1 baked potato equals a fist.

Meat, Chicken, Fish, Dry Beans and Peas, Eggs, and Nuts

- 3 ounces lean meat, chicken, or fish equals a deck of cards or a check book.
- 2 Tablespoons of Peanut Butter equal a Ping Pong ball.

Dairy

- 1 ounce cheese equals about 4 dice.
- 1-½ ounces of cheese equal the size of a 9-volt battery or 3 dominoes.
- ½ cup of ice cream equals ½ baseball.

Fats, Oils, and Sweets

- Use sparingly. For a teaspoon of fat, look to the tip of your thumb.
- 1 teaspoon of butter or margarine equals the size of a postage stamp, or the thickness of a pencil.
- 2 Tablespoons salad dressing equals the size of a Ping Pong ball.

RECIPES

We've included the recipes from all of the diets, and added a few extras for variety. Going forward, we're admitting that they are NOT in order. Refer to the Index for page numbers of your favorites.

Tahini Dressing

2 Tablespoons T*ahini* (sesame seed paste)

3 Tablespoons fresh lemon juice

1 large garlic clove, minced and mashed to a paste

1/8 teaspoon cayenne, or to taste

1/3 cup olive oil or water

Combine all ingredients in cruet and shake well to mix. Refrigerate unused portion.

Herbal Vinaigrette

juice of one lime

juice of one lemon

1/8 to ¼ cup water

1/8 to ¼ cup apple cider vinegar

1 clove finely chopped garlic

1 tablespoon finely chopped thyme, parsley, cilantro, and basil

Combine all ingredients in a jar and shake well. Refrigerate unused portion.

SKINNYCHEATS
The Trainers Secrets

Avocado Dressing

1 ripe avocado

1 lemon, juiced

Mash the avocado until smooth, add the lemon juice and mix until a creamy consistency is obtained. Refrigerate unused portion.

Fruit Salad

1 cup seedless grapes

1 cup orange segments

1 large apple, cut-up

1 large pear, cut-up

Toss all ingredients together, chill, and serve on lettuce lined plate.

Garden Salad

2 large tomatoes, chopped

1 large cucumber, chopped

1 small vidalia onion, chopped

¼ red or green bell pepper, seeded, minced

2 Tablespoons chopped fresh parsley

3 Tablespoons fresh squeezed lemon juice

1 Tablespoon olive oil (light)

1 teaspoon garlic salt

1/8 ground black pepper

In a large bowl, combine tomatoes and the next 4 ingredients. In a separate bowl, use a wire whisk to combine lemon juice and the rest of the ingredients. Pour over the veggies. Cover and refrigerate for 2 hours.

Lettuce and Celery Salad

2   Tablespoons red-wine vinegar

1   Tablespoon finely chopped shallot

¼   teaspoon salt

1/8 teaspoon black pepper

3   Tablespoons olive oil

2   Tablespoons hazelnut oil

2   pounds Bibb lettuce (10 small heads), leaves separated

2   cups celery leaves (from 2 bunches celery; both top leaves and inner leaves from tender pale ribs)

Whisk together vinegar, shallot, salt, and pepper in a small bowl, then add oils in a slow stream, whisking until thoroughly blended. Toss lettuce and celery leaves with just enough vinaigrette to coat in a large bowl. Makes 10 servings.

Spinach Salad

Spinach leaves for bed

¼ cup red onion - soaked in juice from a lemon for a half hour

1 Tablespoon chopped avocado

½ tomato, chopped

¼ cup cauliflower

1 Tablespoon sunflower seeds

Combine all ingredients in a large bowl, and top with mixed salad sprouts and Tahini dressing.

Tomato Salad

1 pound ripe juicy tomatoes,

½ clove garlic

1 Tablespoon balsamic or red wine vinegar

2 - 3 Tablespoons olive oil

salt and freshly-ground pepper to taste

1 ounce fresh mozzarella cheese

handful fresh basil leaves

Wash and core tomatoes and cut into thick slices or wedges. Peel the garlic. In the salad bowl or platter you wish to use, rub the garlic, using the tips of a fork, to make a puree. Add the vinegar and oil. Then, add the tomatoes, tossing gently to coat with dressing. Season to taste with salt and pepper. Slice mozzarella and tuck decoratively in and around the tomatoes. Scatter top of salad with basil leaves.

Tuna Salad

1 7-ounce vacuum-packed chunk light tuna

½ cup pre-shredded coleslaw mix

¼ cup finely chopped onion

1/3 cup fat-free mayonnaise

1 teaspoon apple cider vinegar

Freshly ground black pepper

Romaine lettuce leaves and sliced tomatoes for garnish

Combine tuna, coleslaw mix, onion, mayonnaise and cider vinegar in a medium bowl. Sprinkle with freshly ground black pepper. Garnish with tomato slices. Makes 4 servings – watch your portions.

Broccoli Primevera

3 bunches of broccoli

1/3 cup of raw, Tahini

1 garlic clove

¼ cup lemon juice

1/3 cup spring water

2 teaspoons tamari or sea salt

½ cup chopped mushrooms

½ cup sunflower seeds

¼ cup red onion, chopped

Cut broccoli florets from the stalks and place the florets in a large mixing bowl. Next, blend the Tahini, garlic, lemon juice, water and tamari or salt substitute. Blend until smooth and creamy. Pour the mixture onto the broccoli florets and mushrooms and stir until evenly covered with sauce. Sprinkle in sunflower seeds and onion and stir again. Makes 2-3 cups

Marinated Veggie Kabobs

1 medium eggplant

2 small zucchini

1 or 2 red or green bell peppers

8 medium button mushrooms

2-4 small-medium yellow onions

¼ cup cider or balsamic vinegar

1 tablespoon spicy brown mustard

½ teaspoon rosemary

2 or more cloves garlic chopped

salt and pepper to taste

Wash and cut the vegetables into chunks about 1 inch thick. Place the chunks into a large bowl. In another bowl, combine the vinegar, mustard, rosemary, garlic, and salt and pepper and whisk into a uniform liquid. Pour this liquid over the vegetables and turn the ingredients to ensure each piece is well coated. Cover with plastic wrap and marinate in refrigerator overnight.

Portobello Mushroom Sandwich

4 Portobello mushrooms, sliced into ½ inch slices

1 Vidalia onion, cut into ¼ inch slices

Marinate for a half hour to overnight in:

1 cup soy sauce

juice of one lime

3-4 cloves of garlic, minced

1" piece of ginger root, grated fine

Grill vegetables until done, layer on a crusty roll, and sprinkle with fat-free parmesan cheese

Sprout Salad

1 cup any sprouts (alfalfa, lentil, sunflower, etc)

1 cucumber, diced

2-3 scallions, chopped

3 Tablespoon lemon juice

2 Tablespoons Tahini

1 clove garlic

Pinch cayenne pepper

Put the salad ingredients in a serving bowl. In a small bowl mix the lemon juice, tahini, and garlic minced with the salt. Add pinch of cayenne. Whisk together well. Pour dressing over salad and toss to blend flavors.

Carrot-Sprout Salad

1 cup sprouts, whatever kind you have handy

2 cups grated carrots

¼ cup parsley, finely chopped

3 Tablespoons lemon juice

2 Tablespoons olive oil

pinch cayenne pepper

Put salad ingredients in serving bowl. Blend dressing ingredients in small bowl. Use wire whisk to blend.

Toss dressing and salad and let sit 20 minutes before serving.

French Toast

2 slices of EarthGrain's Honey Almond Oatberry

Bread

¼ carton of Egg Beaters

salt and pepper (to taste)

4 Tablespoons of Light Whipped Topping,

½ cup of fresh or frozen strawberries or

blueberries

1 - 4 Packs of Splenda OR Equal

Non Stick Cooking Spray

Powdered Sugar

Dip each slice of the bread into salted/peppered Egg Beater batter. Toast both sides of bread over medium heat until golden and crisp.

As your toast is cooking, place strawberries into the microwave in a microwaveable dish and cook on medium for 1 minute. Next, remove and place one piece of toast on a serving plate.

Place slightly frozen topping in a bowl and VERY GENTLY blend in 1 Tablespoon of the berries and 1 or 2 packs of Splenda or Equal. GENTLY spoon mixture on top of the slice of toast.

Place the other piece of toast on top of the topping mixture. Reserve 1 Tablespoon of the topping. Pour the mixture on top of the assembled toast. Next, spoon on the remaining 1 Tablespoon of topping. Dust with powdered sugar.

Amazing Vegetable Soup

1 cup finely diced celery

1 cup diced onions

1 (28 ounce) can diced tomatoes

2 (10 ounce) cans chicken broth

3 cups water

2 cloves minced garlic

1 cup frozen green beans

1 package taco seasoning mix

Sauté celery and onion using cooking spray. Add tomatoes, soups and water. Add taco mix and garlic. Let simmer partially covered for about 1 hour. Add green beans and simmer another 15 minutes.

Top with Parmesan or other low-fat cheese and a dollop of fat-free sour cream. Watch your portions!

Pesto Soup

½ cup chopped tomato

1/3 cup finely chopped onion

1 small clove garlic, chopped

½ cup shredded carrot

½ cup shredded beet

¼ cup pine nuts

¾ cup fresh basil, loosely packed

1 Tablespoon raw apple cider vinegar

2 to 3 cups water (as necessary)

Fresh basil leaves for garnish

Combine all ingredients in blender or food processor, and process until finely chopped but not smooth. Divide among serving bowls. Garnish with basil leaves if desired. Makes 6 servings.

Gazpacho Orange Soup

½ large tomato – chopped

½ lemon juiced

¾ cup carrot juice

1Tablespoon olive oil

¼ teaspoon oregano

¼ teaspoon basil

2 cloves garlic

1/3 cup pecans

Combine all ingredients in blender, add grated beet, grated zucchini and chopped parsley or red pepper. Blend well, and serve chilled.

Asparagus Soup

2 cups fresh asparagus

1 stick of celery

2 Tablespoons minced parsley

2 teaspoons onion

1 teaspoons olive oil

2 cups hot water

Combine 1 cup hot water and ½ cup walnuts in large pot. Add olive oil, onion, parsley, celery, and asparagus. Bring to boil, then add remaining water. Cover and remove from heat.

Spinach Soup

¼ apple juiced

1 large bunch of spinach

½ tomato chopped

1 small cucumber, peeled and sliced

¼ cup walnuts

Put all ingredients in blender and blend on chop mode. Resulting mixture should be fairly thick. If it is too thin, add more spinach. Heat mixture on medium heat. Serve when thoroughly warm.

Coleslaw

3 cups Grated Carrots

1 cup grated beets

3 cups grated white cabbage

¼ cup chopped parsley

Marinate all ingredients in:

½ cup olive oil

½ cup lemon juice

1 teaspoon honey

1-2 garlic cloves

Refrigerate until cool, then serve.

Chicken Salad

2 cups chopped cooked chicken

1 cup chopped celery

1 clove minced garlic

1 Tablespoon soy sauce

1 Tablespoon olive oil

1 teaspoon vinegar

salt and pepper to taste

Combine chicken, celery, and garlic in bowl. Add soy sauce, oil, vinegar and salt; toss lightly and serve.

Silken Fettucini Alfredo Sauce

9-½ ounces silken tofu (½ package)

1/3 cup Tahini paste

1/3 cup lemon juice

1/3 cup nutritional yeast flakes

3 Tablespoons tamari or soy sauce

basil to taste

fresh pepper to taste

1/8 teaspoon turmeric

Put all ingredients in a blender and blend until smooth. Then, stir sauce into a pot of cooked pasta and warm everything up over medium heat. Top with alfalfa sprouts if desired.

Broccoli soup

4 cups broccoli florets

4 cups nonfat milk

1 can fat-free condensed milk

2 medium chopped yellow onions

2 cloves minced garlic

1 teaspoon salt

1 teaspoon pepper

½ teaspoon ground nutmeg

1 Tablespoon parsley

1 teaspoon basil

1 teaspoon ground sage

2 Tablespoons cornstarch

In a large saucepan, bring milk and condensed milk to a simmer, over med-low heat. Stir constantly to avoid scalding. Add basil, sage, nutmeg, salt to taste, pepper, garlic, and onion.

Place cornstarch in a bowl and add about 3-4 Tablespoons of hot milk and stir until smooth. Slowly pour the cornstarch mixture into the soup, stirring constantly, until you like the thickness. If you accidentally make it too thick, just add more milk. If the cornstarch gets lumpy, use a whisk.

Add the broccoli and let the soup simmer, still stirring, for about 10 minutes.

Low-fat Hummus

1 can garbanzo beans drained, save juice

3 teaspoons lemon juice

3 cloves garlic peeled

2 Tablespoons sesame tahini

½ teaspoon salt

¼ teaspoon pepper

pepper sauce, as desired

Add all ingredients to food processor, process until smooth, add reserved juice and mix to attain a spreadable texture. Season to taste and serve with chips, bagel chips, pita crisps, or veggies.

Makes 6 servings – watch your portions!

Pasta with Tomato, Basil, and Ricotta

1-½ cups tomatoes, chopped

¼ cup fresh basil, chopped

1 tablespoon red onion, minced

1 clove garlic, chopped

½ cup part-skim ricotta cheese

1 tablespoon olive oil

salt and freshly ground black pepper

½ pound, Rotelle, Ziti, Penné pasta, cooked al dente

Combine the tomatoes, basil, onion, and garlic. Stir in the ricotta, olive oil, salt and pepper to taste. Toss hot pasta with the sauce and serve at once.

Salad Nicoise

1 head iceberg, red leaf or butter lettuce

1 (7-ounce) can water-packed tuna

½ pound green beans, cooked

1 small onion, or ½ red onion, sliced

1 tomato, sliced

½ green pepper, seeded and cut in strips

½ red pepper, seeded and cut in strips

2 hard-boiled egg whites, sliced

2 small potatoes, boiled, skinned, and sliced

Low calorie oil free Italian dressing

Parmesan cheese

Wash lettuce and dry in a lettuce dryer or with paper towels. Tear each lettuce leaf in half; line a salad bowl with the leaves.

Drain tuna, flake with a fork, and place around the bowl on the lettuce. Then add each of the ingredients in turn. Mix the whole salad with just enough dressing to coat but not soak the ingredients. Makes up to 4 portions.

Fresh fruit salad

8 cups cut-up mixed fresh fruit (selections can include: oranges, apples, bananas, pears,

peaches, strawberries, raspberries, blueberries, and grapes)
Bibb lettuce

Line a large salad bowl with Bibb lettuce leaves. Fill salad bowl with fruit. Accompany with Poppy Seed Fruit Salad Dressing (see below). 6 to 8 servings.

Poppy Seed Fruit Salad Dressing

¾ cups sugar

1-½ teaspoon onion salt

1 teaspoon dry mustard

1/3 cup vinegar

1 cup canola or olive oil

1 Tablespoon poppy seeds

In a small bowl, combine sugar, salt, and dry mustard. Stir in vinegar. Beat at medium speed while gradually adding oil. Beat 5 to 10 minutes longer, until thickened. Add poppy seeds. Pour into a screw-top jar. Cover tightly and shake vigorously to blend well. Store covered in refrigerator. Shake well before using. Serve on fresh fruit salads, grapefruit sections, or on lettuce wedges. About 1-2/3 cups.

Spicy Veggie Chili

Put four level tablespoons of brown rice on to boil – this will take about 40 minutes to cook while you make the chili.

1 Tablespoon olive oil

1 chopped onions

2 finely chopped carrots

4 garlic minced cloves

1 chopped red bell pepper

1 chopped green bell pepper

2 Jalapeño peppers

2 Tablespoons chili powder

1 teaspoon cumin

1 cup cooked kidney beans

1 cup cooked pinto beans

1 (28-ounce) can chopped tomatoes (save juice)

1 teaspoon salt

½ teaspoon fresh ground black pepper

2 tablespoons fresh cilantro – finely chopped

Warm the oil over low heat in a large pot. Add the onion, carrot, garlic, red and green peppers, and Jalapeños. Cover the vegetables and cook until they are very soft, about 10 minutes.

Remove the lid, add the chili powder and cumin, and cook an additional 2 to 3 minutes, stirring occasionally. Add the beans and the tomatoes and their juice. Increase the heat to medium and bring the chili to a simmer, cook for 20 minutes. Stir in the salt, pepper, and cilantro.

Steak Fajita

1 pound of flank or skirt steak

1 large yellow onion, peeled and sliced with the grain

2 large bell peppers, sliced lengthwise into half-inch wide strips

Marinade:

Juice of 1 lime

2 Tablespoons of olive oil

2 cloves garlic, peeled, minced

½ teaspoon ground cumin

½ fresh Jalapeño pepper, finely chopped

¼ cup chopped fresh cilantro, including stems

Mix all marinade ingredients and pour over steak. Leave steak in the marinade for at least an hour, the longer the better.

Heat a large cast iron pan or griddle. Add a teaspoon of olive oil to the pan. Add the steak, frying on each side to desired doneness. Remove from pan and let sit for 5 minutes.

Reduce the pan heat to medium high. Add a little more oil to the pan if necessary. Add the onions, and bell peppers. Cook, stirring frequently, for 5 minutes.

Slice the meat against the grain into thin slices. Serve immediately with shredded low-fat cheese, salsa, shredded iceberg lettuce, lite sour cream, and warm flour tortillas. Makes 4 – 6 portions!

Pork stir-fry

1 cup uncooked rice

SKINNYCHEATS
The Trainers Secrets

2 cup water

2 Tablespoon oyster sauce

1 teaspoon sugar

1 chicken stock cube

2 Tablespoon water, extra

17 ½-ounce lean pork stir-fry strips

2 teaspoon cornstarch

1 Tablespoon rice wine or dry sherry (optional)

2 Tablespoon soy sauce

2 Tablespoon peanut oil, divided

2 garlic cloves, chopped

1 piece of ginger (½-inch), chopped

1 small red chili pepper (to taste), seeded and sliced

6 spring onions, cut into bite-sized pieces

6-½ ounces snow peas, halved

Wash and steam rice. In medium sized bowl, mix oyster sauce, sugar, stock cube and water together. Combine pork with cornstarch, rice wine, soy sauce and marinate for 10 minutes.

Heat wok or skillet until hot. Add a drizzle of oil (about 1 tablespoon). Stir fry garlic, ginger and chili pepper until fragrant. Stir-fry pork in 1 to 2 batches for about a minute and remove from pan

Add a little more oil (about 1 Tablespoon) to the pan. Stir-fry spring onions and snow peas for 30 seconds until hot, but still crisp. Return pork to pan.

Push pork and vegetables to the side. Mix and add sauce mixture to the pork-vegetable mixture. Stir and bring to a simmer. Mix together and heat through. Serve with steamed rice.

Vegetable Satay

¼ cup soy sauce

2 Tablespoons rice wine vinegar

1 Tablespoon minced ginger

1 teaspoon minced garlic

2 Tablespoons olive oil

1 teaspoon toasted sesame oil

1 teaspoon brown sugar

Pinch cayenne

4 whole Shiitake mushrooms

4 round zucchini slices, cut ¾-inch thick

4 round yellow squash slices, cut ¾ -inch thick

4 half moon eggplant slices, cut ¾-inch thick

4 pearl onions, halved

4 cherry tomatoes, halved

Soak 8-inch wooden skewers in warm water for at least 45 minutes before using. In a small bowl combine soy sauce, vinegar, ginger, garlic, oils, brown sugar, cayenne and ¼ cup water. Thread vegetables on skewers and place in a shallow glass-baking dish. Pour soy sauce mixture over and marinate skewers, turning several times, for at least 1 hour at room temperature. Preheat grill. Place skewers on grill and cook, turning and basting frequently with extra marinade, for about 6 minutes in all.

Honey Mustard Pork Chops with Sweet Potato

2 Tablespoon. Dijon mustard

1 Tablespoon. peanut oil

2 teaspoons honey

4 pork loin chops, ¾ inch thick

In small bowl stir together mustard, oil and honey; set aside. Place chops on rack of broiler pan. Broil 4 inches from heat source 8 minutes. Brush with half the sauce. Broil 2 minutes longer. Turn chops and broil 8 minutes. Brush with remaining sauce. Broil 3 to 5 minutes longer or until tender and browned.
Meantime, cut a medium-large sweet potato into one-inch thick slices, brush with a little olive oil and grill for five to seven minutes, turning once. Serve the pork chops and grilled sweet potato slices with lots of crisp salad. Makes 4 servings – watch your portions!

Turkey Frittata Florentine

4 slices turkey bacon, cut up

½ cup chopped onion

1 clove garlic, chopped

1 teaspoon butter

1 (10 ounce) package. frozen spinach, thawed and well drained

½ cup chopped tomato

2 (8 ounce) cartons Egg Beaters

½ cup low fat cottage cheese

In 10-inch nonstick ovenproof skillet, over medium-high heat, cook bacon, onion and garlic in butter until tender. Stir in spinach; cook 1 minute more. Stir in tomato. Remove from heat.

In large bowl, beat egg product and cottage cheese until foamy, about 3 minutes. Pour over vegetable mixture in skillet. Bake at 375 degrees for 20 to 25 minutes or until set. Serve immediately. Makes 6 servings – watch your portion size.

Salmon Pasta

½ cup Canola oil

6 cloves garlic, finely chopped

½ cup chopped onion

1 pound bow tie pasta

3 Tablespoons fresh lemon juice

½ cup chopped scallions

¼ cup chopped Italian parsley (plus more for garnish)

½ pound sliced smoked salmon slices

Salt and Pepper

Thin lemon slices for garnish

Heat the oil in a skillet over low heat; add the garlic and onion. Cook until the garlic and onion are soft. Set aside. Cook the bow tie pasta and drain well. Put the pasta back in the pot it was cooked in. Add the garlic and onion mixture and mix well. Add the lemon juice, scallions, parsley, and salmon, and mix well again. Season with salt and pepper to taste. Garnish with Italian parsley and lemon slices, if desired.

Goulash

2 pounds skinless ground chicken breast

½ cup chopped bell peppers

½ cup chopped onions

1 cup shredded low-fat mozzarella cheese

26 ounces low-fat spaghetti sauce

8 ounces uncooked elbow macaroni

1 cup water

1 teaspoon salt

½ teaspoon black pepper

Preheat oven to 350°. Prepare a 13"x 9" casserole dish with cooking spray; set aside. Cook chicken, bell peppers, and onions over medium-high heat until chicken is no longer pink. Add spaghetti sauce, salt, black pepper, macaroni, and water. Cook until macaroni is tender. Place mixture into prepared dish and bake, covered, for 25 minutes. Remove from the oven and top with cheese. Return to the oven and bake, uncovered, until thoroughly heated and the cheese has melted.

This recipe makes 12 servings – watch your portion sizes!

Ratatouille

3 Tablespoons olive oil

1 thinly sliced onion

4 cloves peeled and sliced garlic

1 small bay leaf

1 small eggplant, cut into ½ pieces

1 small zucchini, halved lengthwise and sliced

1 shredded red bell pepper

4 chopped plum tomatoes

1 teaspoon salt

¼ cup shredded fresh basil leaves

fresh ground black pepper, to taste

Over medium-low heat, add the oil to a large pan with the onion, garlic and bay leaf. Stir occasionally till the onion begins to soften. Add the eggplant and cook for 8 minutes stirring occasionally.

Stir in the zucchini, red bell pepper, tomatoes, and salt, and cook over medium heat until the vegetables are tender.

Stir in the basil and a few grinds of black pepper. Serve on a bed of Jasmine rice, with crumbled Feta cheese and chopped black olives. This recipe makes 4 – 6 servings – Watch Your Portions!

Chicken-In-Foil

4 12" x 18" sheets of foil wrap

4 skinless, boneless chicken breasts

1 cup chunky salsa

1 cup black beans or dark red kidney beans

1 cup frozen or canned sweet corn kernels

Preheat oven to 450 degrees.

Place one chicken breast in the middle of each sheet of foil wrap. Spoon one fourth of the salsa, black beans and sweet corn on each of the four chicken breasts, and seal each pack by folding the top and side edges twice, leaving enough room for heat to circulate inside.

Place packs on a cookie sheet and cook for 20 minutes. Unseal packs carefully.

Chicken with Peach Salsa

2/3 cup picante sauce

2 Tablespoons lime juice

1 (15-ounce can of drained and diced canned peach halves

1/3 cup chopped red or green bell peppers

2 sliced green onions

½ teaspoon cumin

½ teaspoon chili powder

6 boneless skinless chicken breasts

½ cup low-sugar peach or apricot preserves

Mix 1/3 cup picante sauce, lime juice, peaches, pepper and onions – set aside to serve with chicken.

Mix cumin and chili powder. Sprinkle chicken with cumin mixture. Mix remaining picante sauce and preserves. Grill chicken until done, turning and brushing often with preserve mixture -- discard any leftover preserve mixture.

Serve chicken with peach salsa, rice and a green salad.

Italian Sausage and Potatoes

   1 pound Italian sausages

   3 large baking potatoes

   8 ounces "Lite" Italian salad dressing (Robusto or

   Zesty)

Cut up Italian sausage links into bite sized chunks. Cube potatoes (with skins). Place in baking dish, then add Italian salad dressing over all.

Bake uncovered at 350 until sausage is no longer pink and potatoes are tender, approximately 45-50 minutes. Add a green vegetable or salad to complete your meal.

Quick Start Energy Drink

4 ounces of orange juice, 4 ounces of apple juice and a handful of raspberries into a blender. Blend until smooth.

Smoothies

Tropical Fruit Smoothie

   2 frozen bananas, sliced

   1 8-ounce can crushed pineapple

   1 large mango, chopped

2 kiwifruit

Juice of 1 large orange

1 cup low-fat buttermilk

Combine all ingredients in blender and blend on high until smooth. Serves 4.

Vitality Smoothie

1 chopped banana

1 egg

1 teaspoon of wheat germ

½ teaspoon Brewer's yeast

1 cup skim milk

2 Tablespoons of nonfat yogurt

honey to taste

2 shakes of cinnamon

½ small scoop of ice

Combine all ingredients in blender and blend on high until smooth.   Serves 4

Couscous salad

2 cups cooked whole wheat couscous

1 cup chopped cucumber

1 cup chopped tomatoes

½ cup chopped red onion

1 cup canned garbanzo beans, drained

1/3 cup fresh mint, chopped

Juice of two large lemons

1 Tablespoon olive oil

Combine couscous, cucumber, tomatoes, onion, garbanzo beans and mint in a large bowl. Whisk together lemon juice and olive oil. Pour over couscous salad and stir well. Cover and refrigerate for at least 2 hours.

Aromatic Lamb Chops

1 Tablespoon chopped garlic

1 Tablespoon chopped rosemary

1 Tablespoon chopped shallots

1 Tablespoon balsamic vinegar

1 Tablespoon chopped parsley

1 Tablespoon chopped onion

1 Tablespoon Canola or Olive oil

12 (1 ounce each) rib lamb chops

Salt and pepper to taste

Mix all the ingredients, except the oil and chops, in a large, non reactive roasting pan. Add the lamb chops, cover, and marinate in the refrigerator for 6 hours. Heat a large skillet until a drop of water sizzles in its center, add the oil and the lamb chops, and sauté the chops for 2 minutes on each side for rare meat, 3 minutes for medium-rare meat, and 4 minutes for well-done meat. Serves 4 (3 chops each) for lunch or dinner.

SKINNYCHEATS
The Trainers Secrets

Skinny latte

4 ounces Italian roast espresso, brewed

4 ounces steamed skim milk

4 ice cubes (made of frozen coffee)

Add (sweetened) hot espresso and steamed milk to a tall glass of ice and stir. If desired, sprinkle top with ground cinnamon.

Sweet and Sour Chicken

2 cups instant whole-grain brown rice

¼ cup seasoned rice vinegar

2 Tablespoon lite soy sauce

2 Tablespoon cornstarch

2 Tablespoon canola oil

2 Tablespoon apricot preserves

1 pound chicken breast, cut in bite-size pieces

1 clove minced garlic

2 teaspoons finely grated or minced ginger

1 cup low sodium chicken broth

2 cups broccoli florets

1 cup sliced carrots

1 cup red pepper, chunked

1 cup green pepper, chunked

1 cup snow peas

1 5-ounce can sliced water chestnuts, drained

Prepare rice according to package instructions.

Combine vinegar, soy sauce, cornstarch and apricot preserves in a small bowl. Set aside.

Heat 1 Tablespoon oil in a large skillet over medium-high heat. Add chicken and cook, undisturbed, for 2 minutes. Continue cooking, stirring occasionally, until chicken is no longer pink on the outside and just starting to brown, then transfer to a plate

Add remaining oil, garlic, and ginger to pan and cook, stirring, until fragrant. Add broth and bring to boil, stirring constantly. Add vegetables, reduce heat to a simmer, cover and cook until the vegetables are tender-crisp. Stir in water chestnuts and chicken. Thoroughly mix the reserved sauce and add to the pan. Simmer, stirring constantly, until the sauce is thickened and the chicken is thoroughly heated. Serve with the rice.

Each serving consists of 1-½ cup stir-fry with ½ cup rice – Watch Your Portions!

Salmon with Red Potatoes

1-½ pounds red potatoes, cut into 1-inch chunks

1 Tablespoon olive oil

¼ teaspoon salt

¼ teaspoon pepper

4 (6 ounce) Salmon fillets

2 Tablespoons horseradish

½ cup fresh dill, divided Preheat oven to 450°. In a 15 ½" x 10 ½" pan, toss potatoes with oil, salt and pepper. Roast potatoes in oven for 10 minutes. After

10 minutes, remove pan from oven. With spatula, push potatoes to one end of the pan to make room for the fish.

Place fish in pan, sprinkle with ½ teaspoon salt. Return to oven and continue roasting with potatoes until fish flakes easily and potatoes are brown. If needed, remove the fish and continue roasting the potatoes until done.

Transfer fish to a platter, top with horseradish sauce and half of the fresh or dried dill. Toss potatoes with remaining dill and serve alongside salmon. Serve with steamed green vegetables.

Quick Beef Chili.

2 teaspoon canola oil

2 garlic cloves, crushed

1 cup chopped onion

1 rib celery, chopped

1 red bell pepper, chopped

1 pound extra-lean ground beef

1 28-ounce can diced tomatoes (with jalapenos, if available)

2 Tablespoon tomato paste

1 15-ounce can dark red kidney beans, drained

1 15-ounce can pinto beans, drained

2-3 Tablespoon chili powder, or to taste

1 Tablespoon ground cumin

Heat oil in a large Dutch oven. Add garlic, onion, celery and pepper, and sauté gently for 2-3 minutes. Add ground beef and cook until meat is browned, about 5 minutes.

Add tomatoes, tomato paste, beans, chili powder and cumin.

Chocolate Pudding Cake

2 cups flour

1 cup sugar

½ cup unsweetened cocoa powder

1 Tablespoon AND 1 teaspoon baking powder

¼ teaspoon salt

1 cup nonfat milk

½ cup unsweetened applesauce

2 teaspoons vanilla extract

2 cups boiling water

1-½ cups firmly packed light brown sugar

½ cup unsweetened cocoa powder

•

• Prepare a 13" x 9" x 2" baking pan (use Pam or a similar cooking spray and set aside).

Combine flour, sugar, cocoa, baking powder, and salt in a large bowl, and beat until batter is smooth. Blend in remaining cake ingredients, stirring thoroughly. Pour into baking pan, spreading evenly.

In a large bowl, whisk pudding ingredients together until sugar and cocoa are dissolved, then pour over cake batter – pudding layer will be thin and runny.

Bake for 35-40 minutes, or until top is firm to the touch. Let cake rest for 15 minutes before cutting. Cover and refrigerate leftovers for up to 7 days or wrap tightly and freeze for up to 2 months. This recipe makes 24 servings – watch your portions!

Low Fat Cherry Cheesecake

1   6-ounce reduced fat graham cracker crust

1   21-ounce can of low sugar cherry pie filling

1   cup skim milk

1   package cheesecake flavor instant pudding and pie filling mix

1   8-ounce tub of Cool Whip Free, thawed

Spoon half of the pie filling into crust. In a mixing bowl, combine milk, and pudding mixes, and whip until smooth, folding in whipped topping. Spoon mixture over pie filling. Refrigerate until set. Top with remaining pie filling.

Oatmeal Goodies

3 cups oatmeal

1 cup whole wheat flour

1 teaspoon soda

¼ teaspoon nutmeg

1 cup unsweetened applesauce

¾ cup sugar

1 teaspoon vanilla

2/3 cup raisins (dried apples, or dried cranberries may also be used)

Combine the first four ingredients, then add the next 3 ingredients, stirring well. Stir in dried fruit. Divide the dough into small balls and mash to ¼ " thickness on the cookie sheet. Bake at 275 degrees for 22-25 minutes. Makes about 50 cookies – Watch your portions!

INDEX

SKINNYCHEATS
The Trainers Secrets

Apple Cider Vinegar Diet

Body Mass Index

Body Mass Index Chart

Body Monitor

Cabbage Soup Diet

Citrus Fruit

Chicken Soup Diet

Diet Myths

Diuretics

    Apple Cider Vinegar

    Asparagus

    Beets

    Brussels Sprouts

    Cabbage

    Carrots

    Celery

    Cucumber

Garlic

Horse Radish

Lettuce

Onions

Radishes

Tomatoes

Fat Flush Foods

    Apples

    Berries

    Citrus Fruit

    Fresh Fruit

    Garlic Oil

    Soybeans

Fiber

Grapefruit Diet

Herbs

    Cayenne

    Cordyceps

    Flaxseed

SKINNYCHEATS
The Trainers Secrets

Ginger

St. John's Wort

Oat Straw

Psyllium

Siberian Ginseng

Ice Cream Diet

Lemonade Diet

Love It and Lose It Diet

Metabolism

Portion Sizes

Sacred Heart Medical Diet

Seven Day All-You-Can-Eat Diet

Serving Sizes

Soybeans

The Trainer's Kick Start Diet

Water

Recipes:

Amazing Vegetable Soup

Aromatic Lamb Chops

Asparagus Soup

Avocado Dressing

Broccoli Primavera

Broccoli Soup

Carrot-Sprout Salad

Chicken-In-Foil

Chicken with Peach Salsa

Chocolate Pudding Cake

Couscous Salad

French Toast

(Fresh) Fruit Salad

(Skinny) Fruit Salad

Garden Salad

Gazpacho Orange Soup

Goulash

Herbal Vinaigrette

Italian Sausage and Potatoes

SKINNYCHEATS
The Trainers Secrets

Lettuce and Celery Salad

Low-fat Hummus

Lower Fat Cherry Cheesecake

Marinated Veggie Kabobs

Oatmeal Goodies

Pasta with Tomato, Basil, and Ricotta

Pesto Soup

Pork Stir-fry

Portobello Mushroom Sandwich

Quick Beef Chili

Ratatouille

Salad Nicoise

Salmon with Red Potatoes

Salmon Pasta

Skinny Latte

Spicy Veggie Chili

Spinach Salad

Spinach Soup

Sprout Salad

Steak Fajita

Sweet and Sour Chicken

Tahini Dressing

Tomato Salad

Tuna Salad

Turkey Frittata Florentine

Vegetable Satay

RESOURCES

From mothers to daughters: transgenerational food and diet communication in an underserved group. Journal of Cultural Diversity, Spring, 2004 by Diane Baer Wilson, Catherine Musham, Mary S. McLellan

Dietary Guidelines for Americans 2005. Washington, DC: U.S. Department of Health and Human Services U.S. Department of Agriculture; 2005. HHS Publication number: HHS-ODPHP 2005-01-DGA-A.

Fitness: Theory and Practice: The Comprehensive Resource for Fitness Instruction. Aerobics & Fitness Association of America; 4th edition (2002).

Nutrition and Diet Therapy Dictionary by Rosalinda T. Lagua, and Virginia S. Claudio. Blackwell Publishing Professional; 5 edition (2004).

A Prescription for Nutritional Healing by James F., M.D. Balch, Phyllis A., C.N.C. Balch. Avery Books (2006).

The Ultimate Fit or Fat, by Covert Bailey. Houghton Mifflin (2000)

Perspectives in Nutrition by Gordon M. Wardlaw and Jeffrey Hampl. McGraw-Hill (2006).

ABOUT THE TRAINERS

Three nationally certified trainers in association with Master Trainer, Ann Macklin, living, working out, and eating in Atlanta GA have come together to combine more than thirty years of exercise and nutritional expertise as they share their secrets to a trim and healthy body.

Areas of training expertise include strength, flexibility, cycling, dance, and endurance. Ranging in age from forty to sixty-four, our trainers not only believe in the truth of wellness and weight control, they believe in sharing how they do it.